Active Living Every Day

SECOND EDITION

Steven N. Blair, PED
Arnold School of Public Health,
University of South Carolina

Andrea L. Dunn, PhD
Klein Buendel, Inc., Golden, CO

Bess H. Marcus, PhD
Department of Family and Preventive Medicine
University of California, San Diego

Ruth Ann Carpenter, MS, RD
Health Integration, LLC

Peter Jaret, MA

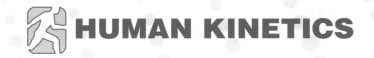

Library of Congress Cataloging-in-Publication Data

Active living every day / Steven N. Blair ... [et al.]. -- 2nd ed.
    p. cm.
  Includes bibliographical references and index.
  ISBN-13: 978-0-7360-9222-7 (soft cover)
  ISBN-10: 0-7360-9222-6 (soft cover)
  1. Exercise. 2. Physical fitness. 3. Health. I. Blair, Steven N.
  RA781.A196 2011
  613.7'1--dc22
                      2010028828

ISBN-10: 0-7360-9222-6 (print)
ISBN-13: 978-0-7360-9222-7 (print)

Acquisitions Editor: Michelle Maloney; **Managing Editor:** Amy Stahl; **Assistant Editors:** Casey A. Gentis, Rachel Brito; **Copyeditor:** Alisha Jeddeloh; **Indexer:** Betty Frizzéll; **Permission Manager:** Dalene Reeder; **Graphic Designer:** Keri Evans; **Graphic Artist:** Dawn Sills; **Cover Designer:** Keith Blomberg; **Photographer (cover):** Neil Bernstein; **Photographer (interior):** Human Kinetics, unless otherwise noted. Photos on page 16 © Marka/Photoshot; pages 20, 124 © Cultura/Photoshot; pages 30, 42, 66, 67, 79, 134 © PA Photos; pages 46, 71, 128 © Photoshot; page 77 © David Herrod/Image State/age Fotostock; page 96 © W. Ron Sutton, President, Accusplit; **Photo Asset Manager:** Laura Fitch; **Photo Production Manager:** Jason Allen; **Art Manager:** Kelly Hendren; **Associate Art Manager:** Alan L. Wilborn; **Illustrators:** Dick Flood, Keri Evans, and Roberto Sabas; **Printer:** United Graphics

Printed in the United States of America   10 9 8

The paper in this book is certified under a sustainable forestry program.

Human Kinetics
1607 N. Market St.
Champaign, IL 61820
Website: www.HumanKinetics.com

In the United States, email info@hkusa.com or call 800-747-4457.
In Canada, email info@hkcanada.com.
In the United Kingdom/Europe, email hk@hkeurope.com.

For information about Human Kinetics' coverage in other areas of the world,
please visit our website: **www.HumanKinetics.com**

E5122

Tell us what you think!
Human Kinetics would love to hear what we
can do to improve the customer experience.
Use this QR code to take our brief survey.

Contents

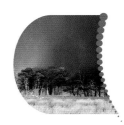
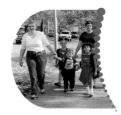
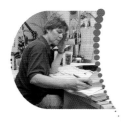
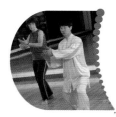
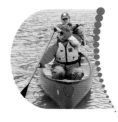

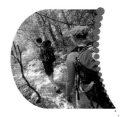

Chapter Twelve: Making Lasting Changes

Celebrating your accomplishments, discovering ways to renew your motivation to remain active, and troubleshooting problems so that you remain on track

Foreword

People in Western societies are becoming increasingly more sedentary. We sit in front of televisions and computers for endless hours. We rarely transport ourselves to work or school by walking or riding bicycles. We gravitate to elevators and escalators to avoid climbing stairs. Our occupations involve far less physical activity than they once did. And relatively few of us routinely engage in planned exercise. One result of these trends is the obesity epidemic. But obesity is only the most visible health problem associated with physical inactivity. Heart disease, cancer, diabetes, and mental health problems occur at much higher rates than they would if most people led physically active lives.

Although the health effects of physical activity are understood now better than ever, the recommendation that we live active lives is far from new. As early as the fifth century BC, Hippocrates recommended regular walking and other forms of moderate activity to promote health and treat illness. In the modern era, prominent health and medical organizations, including the American College of Sports Medicine, American Heart Association, and Centers for Disease Control and Prevention, have recommended regular physical activity for virtually all segments of the population. In 2008, the U.S. Secretary of Health and Human Services released the *Physical Activity Guidelines for Americans,* an extensive research-based document that called on all adults to engage in at least 150 minutes of moderate to vigorous physical activity each week.

One way to accumulate 150 minutes of moderate physical activity in a week is to walk briskly for 30 minutes per day, five days per week. That's not an intimidating or unattainable amount of exercise for the typical person, yet most of us aren't doing it. Some people think they are too busy to be physically active. Others don't know how to get started. Some know how to start but don't know how to maintain an active lifestyle. And some just find the whole idea to be overwhelming.

If one of those statements describes you, or if you're already active but need some new ideas and fresh strategies, this book is for you. *Active Living Every Day* is a tested and proven program for improving your health and well-being through physical activity. It provides information, skills, and a step-by-step process for creating an active lifestyle. Try it and see what a difference physical activity can make in your life. I encourage you to get started today.

Russell R. Pate, PhD
University of South Carolina
Arnold School of Public Health, Department of Exercise Science

You've Come to the Right Place!

By opening this book, you've taken the first important step toward becoming physically active. To make any change for the better, you have to *want* to change. The fact that you're here means you've taken that first step. This program will help you succeed.

There are plenty of good reasons to add physical activity to your life. Something as simple as a half hour of brisk walking every day can make a big difference in your health and how you feel about your life. Pushing yourself a little harder can increase the benefits. Here are some results you can expect:

- More energy
- Brighter mental outlook
- Reduced risk of heart disease, high blood pressure, stroke, and diabetes
- Reduced risk of colon and breast cancer
- Less chance of colds and flu
- Healthy bones, joints, and muscles
- Better weight control
- Maintained fitness and flexibility
- Reduced risk of depression
- Improved sleep quality
- Healthier and longer independent life

If a pill could offer so many benefits, we'd all want to take it, yet more than 50 percent of Americans still aren't active enough for their own good. Why? Because it's easy to be inactive. Labor-saving devices such as cars, elevators, riding mowers, and washing machines have taken over tasks that used to demand physical effort. According to one estimate, most of us burn 700 to 800 fewer calories each day going about our lives than people did just 30 years ago (James et al. 1995).

What can we do? One option is to find time to exercise. Some people can manage to fit in a workout three to five times a week. But not everyone likes to exercise. Many of us are busy with work and family. We barely have enough time in the day to do what we need to do, let alone what we know we should do.

Or so we think.

In fact, there are simple, easy, and enjoyable ways to add activity to your life. Walking instead of driving, climbing the stairs instead of taking the elevator, dancing, and riding a bike all offer good ways to incorporate activity into your lifestyle. Together, they add up to better health, a fitter body, and a potentially longer life.

A Step-by-Step Plan That Works—We Can Prove It

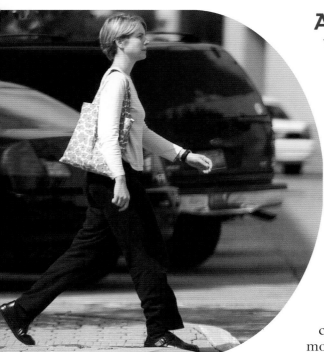

You can find many ways to add physical activity to your daily life.

Most people don't need to be convinced that they should become active. They simply need to learn how to fit physical activity into their lives. That's why we've put together this step-by-step program that is based on scientifically tested methods.

Here's a little background. Beginning in the mid-1950s, exercise scientists focused almost exclusively on the health and fitness benefits of vigorous and sustained exercise. Then work by Dr. Steven Blair and others helped to spark a new way of thinking about physical activity. These studies showed that men and women who were moderately fit had a substantially lower risk for heart disease, stroke, and premature death than those who were unfit and sedentary. The benefits of being moderately fit applied to almost everyone: smokers and nonsmokers, people with high cholesterol or high blood pressure, even those with a family history of early cardiovascular disease. Surprisingly, even obese people who were moderately fit had lower death rates than thin people who were unfit. What mattered was the amount of exercise people did, not how intense the activity was.

With those findings in mind, we designed a study, Project *Active*, to test a lifestyle approach compared with a standard fitness-center approach to increase and maintain physical activity. We recruited 235 men and women who were currently doing little or no exercise. Half of them committed to doing a standard gym workout three to five times a week. The others, part of our lifestyle group, met in small groups to talk about ways to incorporate physical activities such as walking and stair-climbing into their everyday lives.

By almost every measure, men and women in the lifestyle group enjoyed the same benefits as the people who worked out at the fitness center. After two years, their average blood pressures dropped. They lost the same amount of body fat. They were burning the same number of extra calories from activity as the hard-core gym goers. They also gained the same improvements in fitness. For years after our program

Many participants in our program found activities they enjoyed.

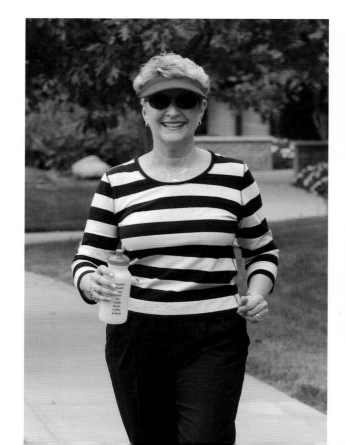

Small lifestyle changes, such as taking the stairs, can greatly improve your health.

ended, many participants were still maintaining an active lifestyle. It seems that many people find it easier to stick with activities that are part of their daily lives rather than gym routines (Dunn et al. 1999).

Our findings showed that almost anyone who is sedentary and unfit can benefit enormously from becoming just moderately fit through physical activity. That's great news. It means you can gain the benefits of physical activity at the gym *or* on your own.

To make active living available to people everywhere, we transformed the research materials from Project *Active* into the Active Living Every Day (ALED) program. Over 34,000 copies of the book have been sold worldwide. Most of the books have been used in ALED programs delivered by 175 nonprofit organizations, corporations, public health departments, health care groups, and research institutions. Research studies using ALED have shown that it

- helps older adults increase their physical activity (Wilcox et al. 2008),
- helps people with arthritis become more active (Callahan et al. 2007),
- can be successfully implemented using an Internet format to increase physical activity and reduce cardiovascular risk among overweight adults (Carr et al. 2008), and
- helps people maintain their new, higher physical activity level for at least six months (Wilcox et al. 2008) and as long as two years (Dunn et al. 1999).

For these reasons, our program can help almost anyone become more active.

Making a Change for the Better

We've based this book on the latest psychological research about behavior change and our experiences using the program. But we've gone a step further. The original Project *Active* program lasted 20 weeks. More recently we tested a shorter 12-week version of the same program. It proved to be just as effective in helping people make lasting physical activity changes. This revised edition of ALED is based on a 12-session program. We think it will appeal to more people and thus encourage more people to become active.

Thanks to feedback from our volunteers, we were able to create a program based on what people need, want, and enjoy. We saw what worked and what didn't. From our participants' experiences, we've put together one of the first scientifically tested programs for increasing lifestyle physical activity. Unlike many other programs, ours

- considers your readiness to change behavior,
- emphasizes moderate-intensity activities,
- helps you increase the intensity of your activities if you wish,
- lets you create your own activity plan,
- helps you solve problems and overcome obstacles,
- concentrates on activities you can add to your daily routine, and
- gives you tips for making other healthy changes in your life.

How to Use This Book

Making lifelong changes takes time and commitment, but it can happen. Before you get started, a few simple tips can help you get the most out of this book.

1. Take One Step at a Time

It's natural to want to rush in and make big changes all at once, especially when you've made up your mind to become more active. However, plenty of studies have shown that the best way for most of us to make lasting changes is one step at a time, experimenting until we find what works for us. That's why we encourage you to follow the steps in each chapter.

2. Go at Your Own Pace

We designed this book for you to go through one chapter each week. You may end up going through one chapter quickly and another more slowly. All we ask is that you go through each chapter completely and fully apply the skills you are learning. As you increase your everyday physical activities, you may find you want to do more. For example, you may want to go for a longer walk than usual, or you may want to do something more vigorous than a walk. Go for it. The more you do, the better off you'll be. If you get bogged down and need a refresher, feel free to return to a previous chapter. Our participants often found that they learned something new or improved their understanding by reviewing material from earlier in the program.

3. Track Your Progress

Throughout this book, we ask you to write down information. It's important to keep track of your progress so you'll know where you started and what you've achieved. You may also want to buy a pocket-sized notebook to keep with you during the day so you don't have to lug the book around. Later we'll talk about step counters—nifty

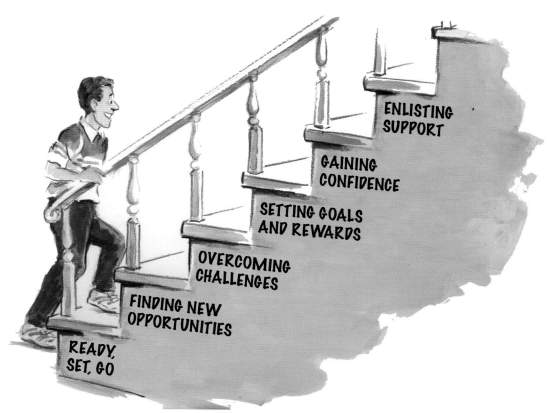

devices that can help you track your progress. For many of our participants, step counters were tremendously helpful.

4. Check Out the Active Living Every Day Online Web Site

 The ALED Online Web site (www.activeliving.info) offers supporting resources for each chapter in the book. Whenever you see this icon in the left margin in this book, you'll find on the ALED Online Web site more in-depth information on topics addressed in the chapter, links to related Web sites, downloadable forms, and resources that will supplement the information in the chapter.

To help you along your ALED journey and make this book simple to use, we've added signposts:

Activity Alerts spotlight the activities we'd like you to do in each chapter.

 Myth Busters debunk some common misconceptions about physical activity and lifestyle changes—misconceptions that get in the way of you becoming active.

 Real Life offers composite sketches of people who have successfully adopted active lifestyles.

Did You Know? offers surprising facts about physical activity and its benefits, many of which include the latest research findings from around the world.

Weighing In highlights advice for people interested in achieving a healthy weight.

Congratulations again on picking up this book. We are confident that this book will help you become active, fit, and healthy as it has done for thousands of others. We look forward to helping you become active every day.

Now let's get started!

References

Callahan, L.F., B. Schoster, J. Hootman, T. Brady, L. Sally, K. Donahue, T. Mielenz, and K. Buysse. 2007. Modifications to the Active Living Every Day (ALED) course for adults with arthritis. *Preventing Chronic Disease* 4(3): 1-10.

Carr, L.J., R.T. Bartee, C. Dorozynski, J.F. Broomfield, M.L. Smith, and D.T. Smith. 2008. Internet-delivered behavior change program increases physical activity and improves cardiometabolic disease risk factors in sedentary adults: Results of a randomized controlled trial. *Preventive Medicine* 46: 431-438.

Dunn, A.L., B.H. Marcus, J.B. Kampert, M.E. Garcia, H.W. Khol, and S.N. Blair. 1999. Comparison of lifestyle and structured interventions to increase physical activity and cardiorespiratory fitness: a randomized trial. *Journal of the American Medical Association* 281(4): 327-334.

James, W.P.T. 1995. A public health approach to the problem of obesity. *International Journal of Obesity and Related Metabolic Disorders* 19(Suppl. 3): S37-S45.

Wilcox, S., M. Dowda, L.C. Leviton, et al. 2008. Active for life: Final results from the translation of two physical activity programs. *American Journal of Preventive Medicine* 35(4): 340-351.

Acknowledgments

The Active Living Every Day program would not have been possible without the hundreds of men and women who participated in our clinical trials that showed that a lifestyle approach to increasing physical activity really does work. We also thank our colleagues at The Cooper Institute and Brown University for their dedication to the successful implementation of the Project *Active* and PRIME research studies. We acknowledge that these studies would not have been possible without the financial support of research grants from the National Institutes of Health.

The second edition of *Active Living Every Day* (ALED) is significantly revised—and we believe, improved—thanks to the nearly 10 years of experience that have ensued since the program was launched. During that time, ALED users gave us feedback on how the program works—or doesn't—in the "real world." We would like to especially thank the many people who were involved in the Robert Wood Johnson Foundation's Active for Life program. We are grateful to members of the Council on Aging of Southwestern Ohio, OASIS Institute, Greater Detroit Area Health Council, FirstHealth of the Carolinas, Jewish Council for the Aging of Greater Washington, the National Program Office at Texas A&M Health Science Center's School of Rural Public Health, and Dr. Sara Wilcox and the evaluation team at the Arnold School of Public Health at the University of South Carolina for their implementation and testing of a 12-session version of the ALED program. Their ideas, experiences, and guidance have led to our decision to release the second edition as a 12-session program.

In addition, we would like to thank our colleagues at Human Kinetics who have shared our passion for helping people attain the many health benefits that a physically active life can offer. Special appreciation goes to Michele Guerra, who guided the initial development of the ALED program to be something much more than this book. Also, the program would not have been sustained over this past decade without Michelle Maloney's management expertise, and we are grateful for her dedication. Finally, we thank Amy Stahl, our editor for the second edition, for her guidance and support.

Steven N. Blair
Andrea L. Dunn
Bess H. Marcus
Ruth Ann Carpenter
Peter Jaret

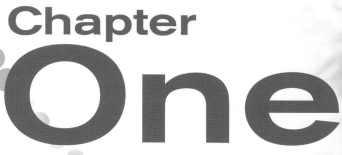

Chapter One

Ready, Set, Go

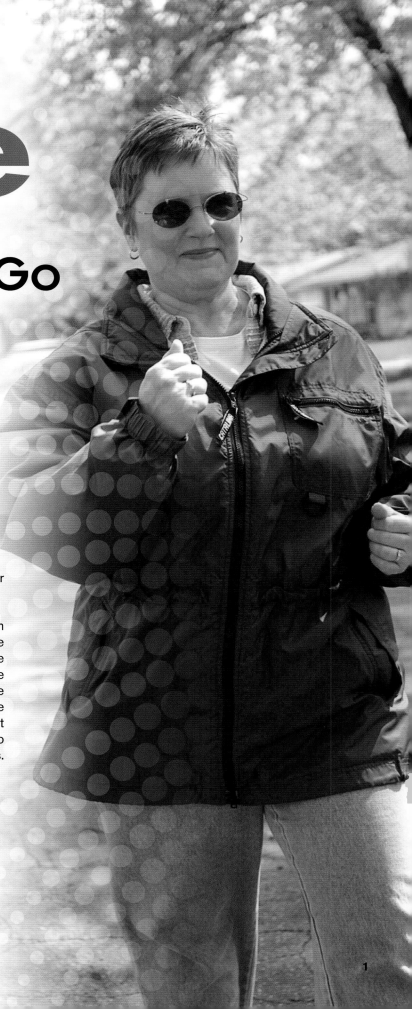

In This Chapter

- Thinking about successful habit changes
- Identifying your readiness for change
- Taking a look at how you spend your time
- Finding time to get up and move
- Assessing the need to check with your doctor before increasing activity

This book was inspired by Project *Active*, our program showing that an active lifestyle can offer most of the benefits of a formal exercise regimen. As exercise scientists, we have always been inspired by the volunteers in our programs, who often overcome obstacles in order to become more active. We'd like to begin by sharing three success stories from Project *Active*. They may inspire you and offer insights into how people successfully change habits and lifestyles.

Real Life

Although Yolanda was retired, she was the primary caregiver to her two young grandchildren. She didn't have much time for exercise. Plus, she had arthritis in her knees, so moving hurt sometimes. Our program showed her that she didn't have to do all her exercise at once to get health benefits. Instead, she could devote the brief segments of time she had each day to fit in 5 or 10 minutes of walking. Eventually she added stairs to her walking routine. After 13 months, she was accumulating 45 minutes of activity at least four days a week. She also began to plan more physical activities to do with her grandkids on the weekend. Yolanda discovered that as she built more strength in her legs, her arthritis pain diminished significantly.

Tommy was on several varsity teams in high school. He stopped playing sports because the community college he went to didn't have athletic teams. As a building-supplies salesperson, he spent a lot of time in the car going between job sites. Occasionally he played a pickup game of basketball. Unfortunately, frequent knee injuries often kept him sidelined. He joined our program at his doctor's recommendation after he was diagnosed with prediabetes. He learned that doing activities at a moderate intensity could lower his risk of advancing to diabetes. That was motivation enough to push him. Tommy learned to think ahead about situations (e.g., injuries, work crises, family time commitments) that might sidetrack his physical activity. He also learned to plan alternative strategies. He cycled instead of ran when he was injured. He walked five minutes at each job site when he couldn't fit in a regular workout. Over time, he found many ways to enjoy his family and be active at the same time.

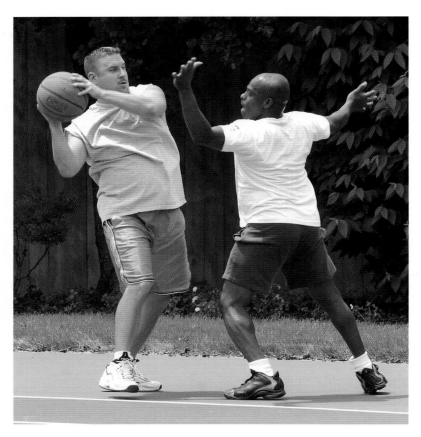

We will show you ways to fit physical activity into your everyday life.

Gwen started the program with the primary intent to lose weight. She had tried all the miracle cures and fad diets, with short-term success and long-term regrets. Even in our program, she got frustrated at first when she didn't lose a lot of weight quickly. We encouraged her to consider the benefits other than weight loss, such as feeling more energetic and more positive about her life. That helped get her through the rough patches. Eventually, by being more active and paying closer attention to her diet, she began to lose weight. Many experts think the slow approach is both healthier and more likely to result in lasting weight loss.

Similar to Yolanda, Tommy, and Gwen, you probably have your own reasons for wanting to be more active. If you're like many of the participants in our program, this isn't the first time you've tried to make a healthy change in your life. Maybe you've quit smoking or cut back on the fat in your diet. Maybe you've started a new hobby or signed up for a course at the community college. Even small changes, such as fastening your seatbelt every time you get in the car or switching from sugary soft drinks to no-calorie beverages, are important. They prove that you can change your habits for the better. This book will help you identify ways you can succeed in living an active life every day. Let's start by looking at habits you have already changed for the better.

 ## Activity Alert

My Personal Successes—Habits I've Changed for the Better

 Take a few minutes now to list one or more of your personal success stories. Think about unwanted habits you've dropped or good ones you've adopted. Then consider why you were able to make a successful change, even a small one. What helped you stick with it? What got in your way? Maybe your biggest obstacle was having enough time, getting distracted during a holiday, or losing your determination. Think about two or three habits you've changed and fill in the following form. You can download a copy of this form from the Active Living Every Day (ALED) Online Web site.

Habits I've changed
1. _____
2. _____
3. _____

Things that helped me succeed
1. _____
2. _____
3. _____

Obstacles that got in my way
1. _____
2. _____
3. _____

From S.N. Blair, A.L. Dunn, B.H. Marcus, R.A. Carpenter, and P. Jaret, 2011, *Active Living Every Day*, 2nd edition (Champaign, IL: Human Kinetics).

By thinking about your past efforts, you can begin to identify some of the things that have helped or hindered your past efforts to make changes for the better. Now let's focus on the process of changing a habit.

Making a Change

Change doesn't happen all at once. It's not a light switch that you can flip on and off. Rather, it is an ongoing process of learning and relearning. Not all of us begin at the same starting point. Researchers have identified five stages of change that most people go through along the way to adopting new habits and behaviors:

1. Precontemplation (not even thinking about a new habit)
2. Contemplation (giving it a thought now and then, but not doing it)
3. Preparation (doing it irregularly)
4. Action (doing the new habit consistently but for less than six months)
5. Maintenance (maintaining the new habit for six months or more)

The point is that change takes place in stages. What's more, progress isn't always in one direction. For every two giant steps forward, there may be one step back. That's normal. You may stay in the stage of contemplation for a long time before you move forward. You may go through the stage of preparation quickly. Then you may stay in action for a short time, stumble, and end up back in preparation. This isn't a sign of failure. It's how change happens.

Skills such as keeping track of your progress and thinking positively can help. In this book we'll help you learn and practice these and other strategies to become physically active for a lifetime.

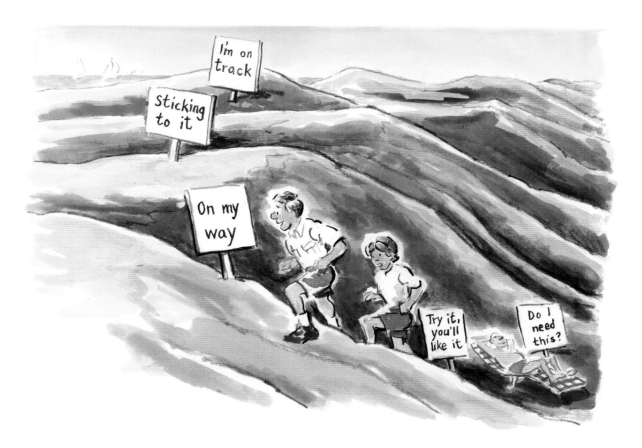

Activity Alert

What's Your Readiness to Change?

Knowing your stage of change can help you discover what you need to do to move forward. The questions in Assessing My Stage of Change will help you gauge where you are on the spectrum between precontemplation and maintenance. In the coming weeks, we'll return to this form to track your progress. You can download a copy of this form from the ALED Online Web site.

Assessing My Stage of Change

Goal: To do physical activity or exercise regularly, such as accumulating

- 150 min of moderate physical activity per week, or
- 75 min of vigorous physical activity per week, or
- a combination of moderate and vigorous physical activity each week, such as
  - a. 75 min of moderate and 40 min of vigorous physical activity, or
  - b. 90 min of moderate and 25 min of vigorous physical activity.

Moderate-Intensity Activity Examples

- Brisk walking
- Biking <10 mph (16 kph)
- Ballroom dancing
- General gardening, such as weeding
- Golfing (no cart)
- Any other physical activity where the exertion is similar to these

Vigorous-Intensity Activity Examples

- Jogging, running
- Tennis
- Biking >10 mph (16 kph)
- Aerobic dancing
- Heavy gardening, such as digging
- Any other physical activity where the exertion is similar to these

Regular physical activity means meeting or exceeding the physical activity goal described above.

For each statement, please mark *yes* or *no*.

1. I am currently physically active (at least 30 minutes per week). ❑ Yes ❑ No
2. I intend to become more physically active in the next 6 months. ❑ Yes ❑ No
3. I currently engage in **regular** physical activity. ❑ Yes ❑ No
4. I have been **regularly** physically active for the past 6 months. ❑ Yes ❑ No

Scoring Key

- *No* to 1, 2, 3, and 4 = **Precontemplation** stage
- *No* to 1, 3, and 4, *Yes* to 2 = **Contemplation** stage
- *Yes* to 1 and 2, *No* to 3 and 4 = **Preparation** stage
- *Yes* to 1 and 3, *Yes* or *No* to 2, *No* to 4 = **Action** stage
- *Yes* to 1, 3, and 4, *Yes* or *No* to 2 = **Maintenance** stage

From S.N. Blair, A.L. Dunn, B.H. Marcus, R.A. Carpenter, and P. Jaret, 2011, *Active Living Every Day*, 2nd ed. (Champaign, IL: Human Kinetics). Adapted from B.H. Marcus and L.R. Simkin, 1993, "The stages of exercise behavior," *Journal of Sports Medicine and Physical Fitness* 33: 83-88. By permission of B.H. Marcus.

Why is it helpful to know your readiness to change? Here are just a few examples.

Let's say you find yourself in the precontemplation stage, which means you're not even thinking about exercise. In that case, becoming aware of the many benefits of activity—and the very real dangers of a sedentary lifestyle—can provide a helpful nudge. Check out appendix B, where you'll find handy references with advice targeted to each stage. For example, the Do I Need This? section on pages 155-156 contains advice for people in the precontemplation stage, including many reasons to become active.

Let's imagine you're in the contemplation stage. You're thinking about being more active, even if you haven't acted on that thought yet. Advice on how to get started can help. Check out the Try It, You'll Like It section on pages 156-157.

Alternatively, let's say you're in the preparation stage. Then you can use tips on overcoming obstacles. Check out the On My Way section on pages 157-158.

You get the idea. The stages of change model can help you know yourself better. It can also point you toward the advice that will be most helpful in moving forward.

❓ Did You Know?

Moderate-intensity activity is equivalent to a brisk walk. How brisk is brisk? The answer depends on many factors, including your health, age, and overall fitness level. The average middle-aged and older adult walking at a moderate-intensity pace would complete a mile (1.6 km) in 15 to 20 minutes. Research studies by us and others have shown that at least 150 minutes per week of any moderately intense physical activity will improve the health and physical and mental functioning of sedentary adults. Studies also show that 75 minutes of vigorous physical activity each week offer the same benefits.

Finding Opportunities to Get Up and Move

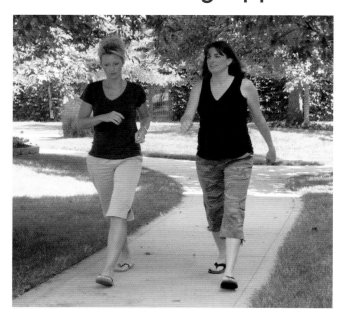

Finding a friend to walk with can help you stay motivated.

What's one of the biggest roadblocks to an active lifestyle? The chair. Many of us are overweight simply because we don't get up and move often enough. We sit in waiting rooms. We sit at desks. We sit in our cars. Of course, there are times when we need to sit. But, there are plenty of other times when we could be moving around instead of sitting. One marketing manager we know at Apple Computer conducts her one-on-one meetings on foot, walking around the company's landscaped grounds. A volunteer for one of our studies made a point of hitting the speaker phone during conference calls and webinars and doing lunges and desk push-ups in her cubicle. A group of people we know at the University of Iowa College of Nursing got together to walk on their breaks.

The point is simple: There are plenty of opportunities for activity. All of us can find time to get up and move between television shows and during commercials, while watching the kids play soccer, during a coffee break, or while we're waiting for the oven to heat up.

Activity Alert

Doing Your Personal Time Study

Most of us have a rough idea of how we spend our time, but few of us know where all those minutes go in our crowded lives. So we're going to ask you to take a close look at how you spend your time. By doing a time study, you'll find opportunities for activity that you might not have known existed.

First, select one typical weekday and one typical weekend day over the next week. Mark them both on your calendar.

Use the Personal Time Study sheet you'll find on page 8 to fill in your activities in four-hour blocks. (Some people like to record their daily routines in one-hour blocks to get a detailed picture of how they spend their time. That's fine. You can use a notepad to break down the time any way you like.)

After you've recorded your activities, determine how many minutes you spend doing any type of physical activity. Also tally up how many minutes you are inactive—sitting, sleeping, driving a car, watching television, or talking on the phone, for instance.

 Throughout this book, we provide many worksheets. Feel free to photocopy them for your use. A few of the forms that you will use the most also appear in appendix D. You can use these extra worksheets for activities you would like to return to when you're struggling to find time to stick to your plan or when problems at home or work are threatening to knock you off track. You can also download the "My Personal Time Study" form from the ALED Online Web site.

Here's what a sample entry might look like.

Date: _____ Day of week: _____			
		Physically active?	
Time slot	**Tasks/activities**	**Yes**	**No**
8:00 a.m. to noon	Desk work		75 min
	Meeting		120 min
	Walk to and from car	7 min	
	Walk to vending machine	3 min	
	Walk to meeting	4 min	
	Talk with coworkers		31 min
	Total time:	**14 min**	**226 min**
Noon to 4:00 p.m.	Walk to lunch room	5 min	
	Lunch		30 min
	Walk back to office	5 min	
	Desk work		180 min
	Walk to lunch room	5 min	
	Coffee break		10 min
	Return to office	5 min	
Total time:		**20 min**	**220 min**

From S.N. Blair, A.L. Dunn, B.H. Marcus, R.A. Carpenter, and P. Jaret, 2011, *Active Living Every Day*, 2nd ed. (Champaign, IL: Human Kinetics).

Personal Time Study

Record your activities for one weekday and one weekend day. Use one sheet for each day. Try to keep this page with you and write things down as you go. Remember to add up the minutes you were physically active and record those in the Yes column. Then add up the minutes you were inactive. The total active and inactive minutes for each four-hour block should be 240. Add up the total number of active and inactive minutes in your day at the bottom of the sheet.

My Personal Time Study

Date: _____   Day of week: _____

Time slot	Tasks/activities	Physically active?	
		Yes	**No**
Midnight to 4:00 a.m.			
4:01 to 8:00 a.m.			
8:01 a.m. to noon			
12:01 to 4:00 p.m.			
4:01 to 8:00 p.m.			
8:01 p.m. to midnight			
	Total time:		

Surprised by how much time you spend sitting? You're not alone. The modern world with all its conveniences has conspired to make life inactive for most of us. In one study (Matthews et al. 2008), researchers tracked the amount of time people were sedentary during waking hours. Children were the least sedentary, yet even they spent about six hours per day seated, reclining, or lying down during their waking hours. Studies of adults recorded an average of over nine hours spent being sedentary. That's two-thirds of their waking time.

It doesn't have to be that way. That's why the Personal Time Study is so useful. Many of your inactive minutes are golden opportunities to become active.

Real Life

Jorge never realized how much time he spent sitting until he completed a Personal Time Study form. Looking over what he did every day—or rather, how little he did in the way of physical activity—sounded the alarm. It made him get serious about turning some of that downtime into activity. It also suggested inactive times that could be turned into opportunities for activity. Jorge wasn't the only one who benefitted. Intrigued by the Personal Time Study, his wife, Teresa, filled one out for herself. With three kids to look after and an office job, she felt as if she never stopped. But when she took a closer look, she realized how much time she spent sitting. She sat in the car while driving the kids here and there. She sat at her desk and in meetings. She sat while she watched the kids at dance practice or piano recitals. About the only time she got up and moved, she realized, was when she was preparing meals. She decided then and there that she was going to have to make some changes.

Did You Know?

Despite the urgings of exercise scientists, nutritionists, and other experts in healthy living, the lifestyles of most Americans have become less healthy over the past two decades. These discouraging findings come from an analysis of data from the National Health and Nutrition Examination Survey (King, Mainous, Carnemolla, and Everett 2009). They show that

- the percent of middle-aged adults with a body mass index (BMI) of 30 or more has increased from 28 to 36 percent,
- physical activity more than 12 times a month has decreased from 53 to 43 percent of middle-aged adults, and
- eating five or more fruits and vegetables a day has decreased from 42 to 26 percent of middle-aged adults.

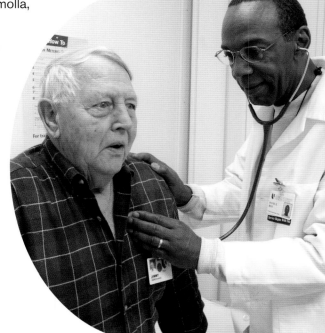

Even though physical activity is good for just about everyone, some people should check with their doctors before doing more physical activity.

Minorities were least likely to follow a healthy lifestyle, the research shows. But the problem cuts across all populations. The findings point out how much work needs to be done to improve health through lifestyle. Unlike other health problems, this one will only be solved if everyone pitches in.

Do I Need a Medical Exam?

In general, moderate-intensity activities are safe. However, if you have serious pre-existing conditions, such as heart disease, diabetes, or cancer, we encourage you to check with your doctor before beginning to exercise even at a moderate intensity. Your doctor may want to give you a medical exam or stress test. If you are sedentary now, we recommend that you don't attempt vigorous activities until you have been doing moderate activities for a while.

Most people following this program are interested in doing moderate-intensity activities. If you want to exercise at a vigorous level, check with your doctor first if any of the following apply:

- You are a man aged 45 or older or a woman aged 55 or older.
- You have *two* or more of the following risk factors: You have high blood pressure, high cholesterol, high blood sugar, or a family history of heart disease; are at least 30 pounds (13.6 kg) overweight; currently smoke; or are not at all active.
- You have heart or blood vessel disease, diabetes, lung disease, asthma, thyroid disorders, or kidney disease.

 ## Activity Alert

Should I See My Doctor?

Fill out the PAR-Q and You questionnaire on page 12 to determine if you are ready to become more physically active. If you answered "yes" to one or more questions, talk with your doctor before you increase your physical activity.

If you answered "no" to all questions, you can increase your activity by beginning slowly and building up gradually—just as we show you in this book. Periodically review this questionnaire and contact your doctor if you answer "yes" to any of the questions.

Now's the Time

In our programs, many participants had never thought about change as a process. They believed that either you change or you don't change. Understanding that there are stages of change provided a useful insight. Many people felt encouraged. We always ask participants how long they have been thinking about increasing their activity. The record? Thirty years! That participant went on to become one of the stars of our program. The moral of the story: It's never too late to get started.

CHAPTER CHECKLIST

Before you move on to the next week's activities, make sure you've done the following:

- Identified at least one habit you have successfully changed
- Filled out the Assessing My Stage of Change questionnaire
- Completed a Personal Time Study for at least two days

- Identified opportunities during the day to add physical activity
- Completed the PAR-Q and You questionnaire and, if necessary, made an appointment to talk with or visit your doctor

 Checked out chapter 1 on the ALED Online Web site for more helpful resources and information for this chapter

References

King, D.E., G. Mainous III, M. Carnemolla, and C.J. Everett. 2009. Adherence to healthy lifestyle habits in US adults, 1988-2006. *American Journal of Medicine* 122(6): 528-34.

Matthews, C.E., K.Y. Chen, P.S. Freedson, M.S. Buchowski, B.M. Beech, R.R. Pate, and R.P. Troiano. 2008. Amount of time spent in sedentary behaviors in the United States, 2003-2004. *American Journal of Epidemiology* 167(7): 875-881.

PAR-Q & YOU

(A Questionnaire for People Aged 15 to 69)

Regular physical activity is fun and healthy, and increasingly more people are starting to become more active every day. Being more active is very safe for most people. However, some people should check with their doctor before they start becoming much more physically active.

If you are planning to become much more physically active than you are now, start by answering the seven questions in the box below. If you are between the ages of 15 and 69, the PAR-Q will tell you if you should check with your doctor before you start. If you are over 69 years of age, and you are not used to being very active, check with your doctor.

Common sense is your best guide when you answer these questions. Please read the questions carefully and answer each one honestly: check YES or NO.

YES	NO		
☐	☐	1.	**Has your doctor ever said that you have a heart condition <u>and</u> that you should only do physical activity recommended by a doctor?**
☐	☐	2.	**Do you feel pain in your chest when you do physical activity?**
☐	☐	3.	**In the past month, have you had chest pain when you were not doing physical activity?**
☐	☐	4.	**Do you lose your balance because of dizziness or do you ever lose consciousness?**
☐	☐	5.	**Do you have a bone or joint problem (for example, back, knee or hip) that could be made worse by a change in your physical activity?**
☐	☐	6.	**Is your doctor currently prescribing drugs (for example, water pills) for your blood pressure or heart condition?**
☐	☐	7.	**Do you know of <u>any other reason</u> why you should not do physical activity?**

If you answered

YES to one or more questions

Talk with your doctor by phone or in person BEFORE you start becoming much more physically active or BEFORE you have a fitness appraisal. Tell your doctor about the PAR-Q and which questions you answered YES.

- You may be able to do any activity you want — as long as you start slowly and build up gradually. Or, you may need to restrict your activities to those which are safe for you. Talk with your doctor about the kinds of activities you wish to participate in and follow his/her advice.
- Find out which community programs are safe and helpful for you.

NO to all questions

If you answered NO honestly to all PAR-Q questions, you can be reasonably sure that you can:
- start becoming much more physically active — begin slowly and build up gradually. This is the safest and easiest way to go.
- take part in a fitness appraisal — this is an excellent way to determine your basic fitness so that you can plan the best way for you to live actively. It is also highly recommended that you have your blood pressure evaluated. If your reading is over 144/94, talk with your doctor before you start becoming much more physically active.

DELAY BECOMING MUCH MORE ACTIVE:
- if you are not feeling well because of a temporary illness such as a cold or a fever — wait until you feel better; or
- if you are or may be pregnant — talk to your doctor before you start becoming more active.

PLEASE NOTE: If your health changes so that you then answer YES to any of the above questions, tell your fitness or health professional. Ask whether you should change your physical activity plan.

<u>Informed Use of the PAR-Q</u>: The Canadian Society for Exercise Physiology, Health Canada, and their agents assume no liability for persons who undertake physical activity, and if in doubt after completing this questionnaire, consult your doctor prior to physical activity.

No changes permitted. You are encouraged to photocopy the PAR-Q but only if you use the entire form.

NOTE: If the PAR-Q is being given to a person before he or she participates in a physical activity program or a fitness appraisal, this section may be used for legal or administrative purposes.

"I have read, understood and completed this questionnaire. Any questions I had were answered to my full satisfaction."

NAME _____

SIGNATURE _____   DATE_____

SIGNATURE OF PARENT _____   WITNESS _____
or GUARDIAN (for participants under the age of majority)

Note: This physical activity clearance is valid for a maximum of 12 months from the date it is completed and becomes invalid if your condition changes so that you would answer YES to any of the seven questions.

CSEP SCPE © Canadian Society for Exercise Physiology   Supported by: Health Canada   Santé Canada   continued on other side...

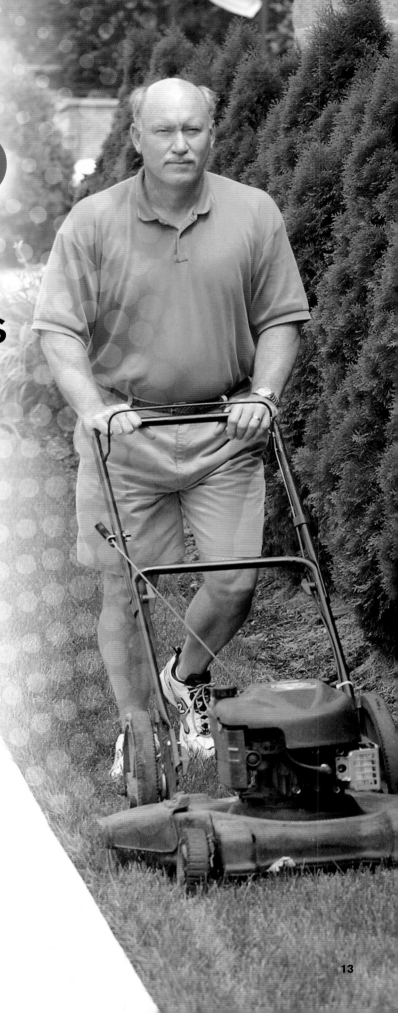

Chapter Two

Finding New Opportunities

In This Chapter

- Taking a two-minute walk
- Turning downtime into opportunities for activity
- Turning light activity into moderate-intensity activity
- Turning moderate-intensity activity into vigorous activity
- Checking out the benefits of walking
- Coming up with an activity plan
- Tracking thoughts about physical activity

Now that you've done your Personal Time Study, you know how much time you spend being active and how much you spend being inactive. In this chapter, you'll find opportunities to turn some of those minutes of inactivity into activity. You'll discover the joys of a two-minute walk. You'll also draw up a plan for adding short walks to your schedule.

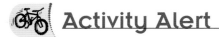

Activity Alert

Take a Walk

We want to begin by asking you to stop reading, put down the book, and hit the road—not for good but just long enough to take a two-minute walk. Go up and down the corridor or block a few times or make a circuit of your house. Use a watch or clock to time yourself. Walk, don't run. And limit your walk to just two minutes. When you're done, come back to this book, and we'll compare notes.

Starting Off on the Right Foot

How did that feel? If it's been a while since you've been active, you may have felt a little winded by the end. Don't worry. If you can walk for 2 minutes, you will soon find that 2 minutes can become 5 minutes, and 5 minutes can become 10 minutes. If you can work up to at least two to three 10-minute brisk walks each day, you'll improve your fitness and get most of the other benefits of physical activity.

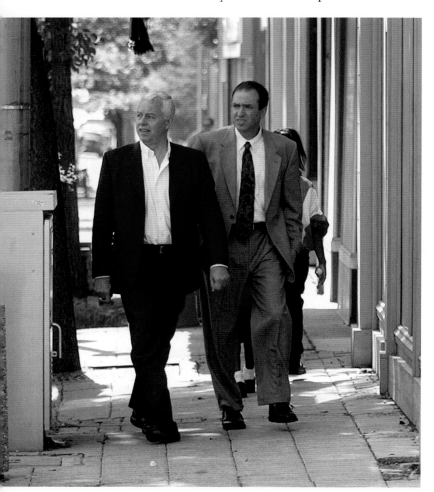

When and where can you take two-minute walks?

The official advice from public health experts in the Physical Activity Guidelines for Americans (Department of Health and Human Services 2008) is at least 150 minutes of moderate-intensity physical activity or 75 minutes of vigorous-intensity activity each week. Keep in mind that you don't have to do it all at once. You can break up the total amount into bouts of 10 minutes or more. You can also do a combination of moderate and vigorous activities to meet these goals, such as walking briskly for 30 minutes on three days and jogging for 15 minutes on two other days.

The two-minute walk is an easy way to build activity into your day without taking a lot of time. You can do it almost anywhere and anytime. Here are a few suggestions:

- Get off the bus one block early and walk the rest of the way to work.
- Walk a block or two for lunch instead of going to the deli right across the street.
- Walk around for two minutes during your coffee break.
- Take a two-minute walk during TV commercials.

Real Life

One of our participants, a computer programmer named Margarita, scheduled three 10-minute walks into her computer. She even programmed it to beep when it was time to take a hike. She used these opportunities to check in on coworkers or grab her mail. Eventually she worked up to accumulating 50 minutes of activity every day. Along the way, she noticed that her energy level and her mood improved. She began to look forward to her day in a way she hadn't before. When she went to the doctor for her annual checkup, she also discovered that her blood pressure was down a few notches, and she'd lost a few pounds, which made her feel even happier.

Activity Alert

Turning Downtime Into Uptime

Look back at your Personal Time Study form on page 8. Using the following form, make a list of each sedentary activity that filled your weekday. Estimate how much time you spent doing each one. You can also download a copy of this form from the ALED Online Web site.

Sedentary activity	Minutes per day
1.	
2.	
3.	
4.	
5.	
6.	

From S.N. Blair, A.L. Dunn, B.H. Marcus, R.A. Carpenter, and P. Jaret, 2011, *Active Living Every Day*, 2nd ed. (Champaign, IL: Human Kinetics).

Surprised by how much time you spent sitting or stretched out on the sofa? Now's the time to change that. Look back at your list and circle one sedentary activity that you can do less of. Logging 90 minutes a day in front of the TV? Shorten that time by getting up and doing something during the commercial breaks. Surprised by how much time you spend on the telephone at home? Walk while you talk using your cell phone or portable phone and a headset. Using the following form, write down your ideas for replacing sedentary activities with more active ones. You can also download a copy of this form from the ALED Online Web site.

1. _____
2. _____
3. _____
4. _____
5. _____
6. _____

From S.N. Blair, A.L. Dunn, B.H. Marcus, R.A. Carpenter, and P. Jaret, 2011, *Active Living Every Day*, 2nd ed. (Champaign, IL: Human Kinetics).

❓ Did You Know?

We're great believers in the benefits of building more activity into everyday life. That's what ALED is all about. We're not the only ones who are excited about this approach. In 2009, researchers at Karolinska University in Sweden published results from a study that encouraged obese middle-aged women to walk or bicycle to work rather than drive or take public transportation. The program worked. After 18 months, commuting by car and public transport dropped by about 35 percent. The change showed in the women's waistlines, which decreased slowly but steadily (Hemmingsson et al. 2009)

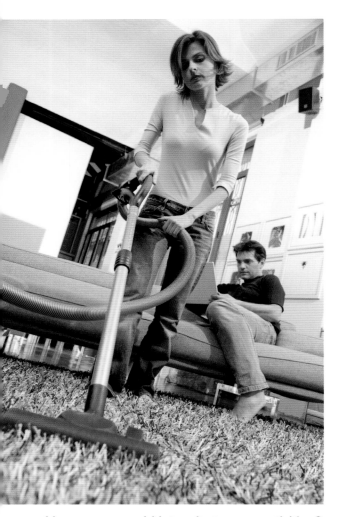

How can you add intensity to your activities?

Turning Light Activity Into Moderate Activity

In addition to increasing the amount of time you are active, you can also increase your daily physical activity by cranking up the intensity. Light-intensity activity is any physical activity more strenuous than sleeping and less strenuous than a brisk walk. Moderate-intensity walking means walking a mile (1.6 km) in 15 to 20 minutes, a pace of 3 to 4 miles (4.8-6.4 km) an hour. It's similar to the way you walk when you're hurrying to make an appointment or to get out of the cold. Vigorous-intensity activities include jogging, riding a bicycle uphill, participating in a strenuous aerobics class, or playing a strenuous sport.

Here are a few simple ways to turn light activity into moderate activity:

- Let's say you usually stroll to the cafeteria on your afternoon break. Instead of walking leisurely, take a brisk walk. You'll turn a light activity into a moderate one. (Go the long way around, and you'll use even more energy.)

- When it's time to vacuum the house, put on your favorite fast dance music and try to keep up. If you feel yourself getting slightly winded, then you're doing moderate-intensity activity.

- Love to shop? First take a fast-paced walk around the mall or shopping area, glancing at what the windows have to offer. Once you've completed your circuit, reward yourself by going back to check out things that intrigued you.

🚲 Activity Alert

Turning Up the Intensity

In the following space, write down two light-intensity activities that you are willing to crank up into moderate-intensity activities simply by picking up the pace.

	Light-intensity activity	How I'll increase it to moderate intensity
1.	_____	_____
2.	_____	_____

From S.N. Blair, A.L. Dunn, B.H. Marcus, R.A. Carpenter, and P. Jaret, 2011, *Active Living Every Day*, 2nd ed. (Champaign, IL: Human Kinetics).

Turning Moderate Activity Into Vigorous Activity

Most of the people in our programs are inactive and want to become more active. Their goal is to move from light to moderate activity levels and meet the guideline in the Physical Activity Guidelines for Americans (Department of Health and Human Services 2008) of 150 minutes per week. But some people are already fairly active and want to push themselves harder. That's great—the more vigorous your activities, the less time it takes to achieve the guideline. If you continue to get 150 minutes per week but at a vigorous intensity, you'll improve your fitness and reap even greater health benefits. Examples of vigorous activities include the following:

- Racewalking, jogging, or running
- Tennis
- Raquetball
- Aerobic dancing
- Bicycling 10 miles (16 km) per hour or faster
- Hiking uphill
- Swimming laps
- Heavy gardening (continuous digging or hoeing)

If you're ready to move from moderate to vigorous intensity, choose an activity that you feel comfortable doing and increase the intensity. For example, if you're comfortable with brisk walking, try jogging or running instead. Start by jogging for just a couple of minutes, and then return to walking briskly. When you're ready, jog again for a couple of minutes. As with any new activity, it's wise to take things slowly, gradually increasing the intensity. In the following space, write down two moderate activities that you are willing to crank up into vigorous activities simply by picking up the pace.

	Moderate-intensity activity	How I'll increase it to vigorous intensity
1.	_____	_____
2.	_____	_____

From S.N. Blair, A.L. Dunn, B.H. Marcus, R.A. Carpenter, and P. Jaret, 2011, *Active Living Every Day*, 2nd ed. (Champaign, IL: Human Kinetics).

Weighing In

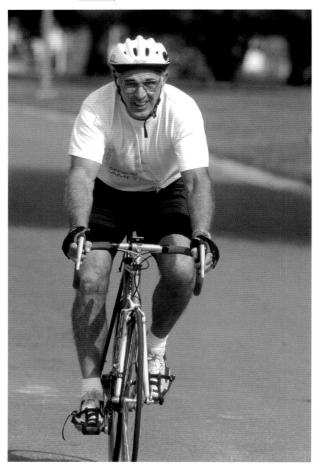

Exercising can help you lose weight and keep it off.

A Word About Weight Control

Americans spend billions of dollars a year on diets and weight-loss plans, yet obesity is rapidly increasing. Why? Because dieting alone doesn't work for most people. Dieters who lose weight typically gain it back. What does work? People who reliably lose weight and keep it off decrease the calories they eat *and* increase the calories they burn through physical activity.

Exercise has a special advantage when it comes to losing weight and keeping it off for good—you don't have to cut back so much on your daily calories. It takes a deficit of 500 calories per day to lose 1 pound (.5 kg) of body fat per week. You can do this by

- eating 500 fewer calories per day,
- eating 250 fewer calories and increasing physical activity by 250 calories per day, or
- increasing physical activity by 500 calories per day.

Most people find it easier to do the second option—reduce calories a little and add a little activity. We think that's the healthiest option, too. It offers the benefits of activity along with the benefits of a reduced-calorie diet that doesn't mean feeling hungry all the time. Most people find it easier to say "yes" three times a day to a brisk walk than "no" many times a day to food. Over time, you can add a little more activity and trim a few more calories from your diet.

 Go to the ALED Online Web site for more information and resources about weight management.

 ## Myth Buster

"I'm just too tired to walk now."

Studies show that being active makes people feel more energetic. There are probably many reasons for this. For one, moving around helps get blood flowing so you feel alert. In addition, many people say they feel better about themselves when they are regularly active than when they are sedentary. They feel more in control, more capable, and more motivated. Moderate exercise increases heart rate and breathing, which can improve overall fitness. The fitter you are, the more stamina you have for physical activity. As you become fit, your body improves its ability to use oxygen, and your heart improves its ability to supply blood to all parts of the body.

One thing you may notice as you become fit is that your heart rate at rest slows down. It takes less effort to pump the same amount of blood to your brain and muscles when you're fit than when you're unfit. A strong heart and cardiorespiratory system mean greater stamina and a decreased chance of heart attack and heart disease.

Walking Works Wonders

Dozens of studies have confirmed the many health benefits associated with walking. Consider a few payoffs:

- **Weight control.** In general, people who successfully lose weight and keep it off incorporate physical activity into their weight-management plan. Even moderate-intensity activities such as brisk walking boost the calories you burn every day.
- **Good health.** Many studies show that walking every day significantly reduces high blood pressure. Surprisingly, moderate activity seems to lower blood pressure better than vigorous exercise.
- **Bright spirits.** Getting up and walking can help fight the blues. Some studies have shown that regular physical activity can help relieve stress and symptoms of depression.
- **High odds of staying healthy.** People who make moderate activities such as walking part of everyday life run less risk of developing heart disease, colon cancer, and other chronic illnesses.

 ## Activity Alert

Coming Up With a Plan

You've given the two-minute walk a try. You've found times during the day when you can get up from your desk or sofa and get moving. Now it's time to commit to a plan. Identify where you can fit in a few two-minute walks this week. During a coffee break is one possibility. During commercials for your favorite TV show is another. Maybe you can park the car at the far end of the lot or get off the bus a stop early and walk the rest of the way. If you're a new parent, you can strap on a baby carrier and take a walk. The goal is to add a little more physical activity to your daily life.

Use a weekly calendar to identify when you will fit in at least one two-minute walk; if you can do more, great. Be specific. Our research shows that the more specific your plan, the more likely you are to follow it.

My Plan for Two-Minute Walks

Monday	
Tuesday	
Wednesday	
Thursday	
Friday	
Saturday	
Sunday	

From S.N. Blair, A.L. Dunn, B.H. Marcus, R.A. Carpenter, and P. Jaret, 2011, *Active Living Every Day*, 2nd ed. (Champaign, IL: Human Kinetics).

❓ Did You Know?

The total number of calories you burn is the same whether you do three 10-minute bouts of activity or one 30-minute session (as long as the intensity remains the same). Finding opportunities for short activities is often easier than finding an uninterrupted half hour. If you're overweight or obese, it may be easier to accumulate shorter bouts during the day. A research group at the University of Pittsburgh found that obese women were more likely to stick with a program of four 10-minute bouts of activity throughout the day compared with one 40-minute bout. The group of obese women who added four 10-minute bouts ended up burning a greater number of calories and tended to lose more weight than the group of obese women who did one 40-minute bout per day (Jakicic et al. 1995).

Two Tips to Help You Stay Motivated

When you're making a big change in your life—whether it's adding activity, losing weight, or quitting smoking—there are times when you may feel discouraged. Don't let that sideline your efforts to change. Here are two simple tips to remember.

1. Lasting changes begin with small steps.

Once you've made up your mind to change, it's natural to want to jump right in and do it. There's nothing wrong with being gung ho. But sometimes people who start with a big bang, end up fizzling before the first lap is over. They buy that gym membership and plunge into a new routine, but by the end of the first week they're so sore and tired they have to take the next week off. Right away they feel discouraged, and soon the gym shoes begin gathering dust in the closet.

We're convinced that for most people, the best way to make a lasting change is to begin gradually. Reward yourself along the way. Have a plan in mind for what you'll do if you don't meet your goal. You'll learn a problem-solving strategy in Chapter Three that will help you devise plans for overcoming obstacles.

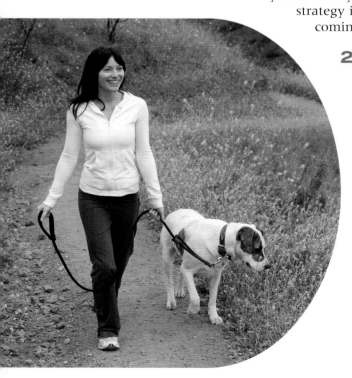

2. Doing something is better than doing nothing.

Adding short stretches of activity during the day can make a difference. You don't have to do your exercise all at once. Doing 10 minutes of moderate-intensity activities three times a day can add up to big health benefits. Every little bit helps. And the longer you stick with your commitment to become more active, the easier it's likely to be. Many of the participants in our program began to discover that they really enjoyed being active. They missed it when something got in the way of their physical activity plan.

It may be easier to accumulate short 10-minute bouts of exercise during the day than to walk a full 30 or more minutes at one time.

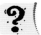

Did You Know?

Any of us who lights up a cigarette these days knows that we're doing ourselves and those around us real harm. We also all know that we'd be better off having a piece of fruit for dessert than helping ourselves to a fat slice of chocolate decadence. But taking the escalator instead of the stairs? Most of us never even pause. We never think, "Uh-oh, if I take the elevator instead of the stairs, I'm likely to raise my risk of heart disease."

However, the cumulative effect of inactivity *is* harmful. The epidemic of inactivity in the United States may be more harmful to our health than an overly rich diet, and it may be just as harmful as smoking. In one study, for instance, we followed over 32,000 people for eight years. People whose only risk factor was low fitness were significantly more likely to die prematurely than those who had high blood pressure, high cholesterol, or a smoking habit but who were at least moderately fit. In other words, moderate fitness—achievable by doing moderate-intensity activities on most days—can help counteract even well-known risk factors for disease (Wei et al. 1999).

Tracking Physical Activity Thoughts

The ability to make a successful change depends a lot on your mental attitude. How you feel about activity—and how you feel about yourself—plays an important role. Keeping track of your thoughts, something psychologists call *self-monitoring*, can be a big help for many people.

The final thing we want you to do in this session is keep track of your thoughts about an active life. Use the self-monitoring form on this page. (A blank copy of this form is located in appendix D on page 166.) Make copies of the form since you'll need to use one each day. You can also download a copy of this form from the ALED Online Web site.

Keeping Track of Thoughts

Instructions: Use this form to record the number of times you think about doing physical activity. Simply place a check mark in a box in section 1 each time you think about doing some physical activity. If you do the activity you were thinking about, place a check mark in a box in section 2.

Keeping track of your thoughts about activity can help you start moving toward an active lifestyle.

Section 1   I thought about doing some physical activity.

☐ ☐ ☐ ☐ ☐ ☐ ☐ ☐ ☐ ☐ ☐ ☐ ☐ ☐ ☐ ☐ ☐ ☐ ☐ ☐
☐ ☐ ☐ ☐ ☐ ☐ ☐ ☐ ☐ ☐ ☐ ☐ ☐ ☐ ☐ ☐ ☐ ☐ ☐ ☐
☐ ☐ ☐ ☐ ☐ ☐ ☐ ☐ ☐ ☐ ☐ ☐ ☐ ☐ ☐ ☐ ☐ ☐ ☐ ☐

Section 2   I carried out my thoughts and did the activity.

☐ ☐ ☐ ☐ ☐ ☐ ☐ ☐ ☐ ☐ ☐ ☐ ☐ ☐ ☐ ☐ ☐ ☐ ☐ ☐
☐ ☐ ☐ ☐ ☐ ☐ ☐ ☐ ☐ ☐ ☐ ☐ ☐ ☐ ☐ ☐ ☐ ☐ ☐ ☐
☐ ☐ ☐ ☐ ☐ ☐ ☐ ☐ ☐ ☐ ☐ ☐ ☐ ☐ ☐ ☐ ☐ ☐ ☐ ☐

From S.N. Blair, A.L. Dunn, B.H. Marcus, R.A. Carpenter, and P. Jaret, 2011, *Active Living Every Day*, 2nd ed. (Champaign, IL: Human Kinetics).

Got a Minute or Two?

With clamoring kids and long commutes, errands to run and people to see, most of us don't have enough time for everything we'd like to do. There's even less time for the things we know we *should* do. But let's be realistic. No matter how busy you are, you can find a few minutes. That's the most important lesson of the two-minute walk. Most commercial breaks on television run longer than two minutes. With all the stations on cable TV these days, it takes longer than that to click through to see what's on. Two minutes is about as long as it takes to heat up water for tea in the microwave. No matter how busy you are, you probably have two-minute stretches of time here and there. We encourage you to use them to do something active.

CHAPTER CHECKLIST

Before you move on to the next week's activities, make sure you've done the following:

- Identified inactive periods during the day that you can turn into activity
- Found at least three ways to turn light activity into moderate activity
- Made a plan for adding a few two-minute walks to your schedule this week
- Started tracking your thoughts about physical activity

 Checked out chapter 2 on the ALED Online Web site for more helpful resources and information for this chapter

References

Department of Health and Human Services. 2008. *Physical activity guidelines for Americans.* Washington, DC: Government Printing Office.

Hemmingsson, E., J. Uddén, M. Neovius, U. Ekelund, and S. Rössner. 2009. Increased physical activity in abdominally obese women through support for changed commuting habits: a randomized clinical trial. *International Journal of Obesity* 33(6): 645-652.

Jakicic, J.M., et al. 1995. Prescribing exercise in multiple short bouts versus one continuous bout: effects on adherence, cardiorespiratory fitness, and weight loss in overweight women. *International Journal of Obesity* 12(12): 893-901.

Wei, M., et al. 1999. Relationship between low cardiorespiratory fitness and mortality in normal-weight, overweight, and obese men. *Journal of the American Medical Association* 282(16): 1547-1553.

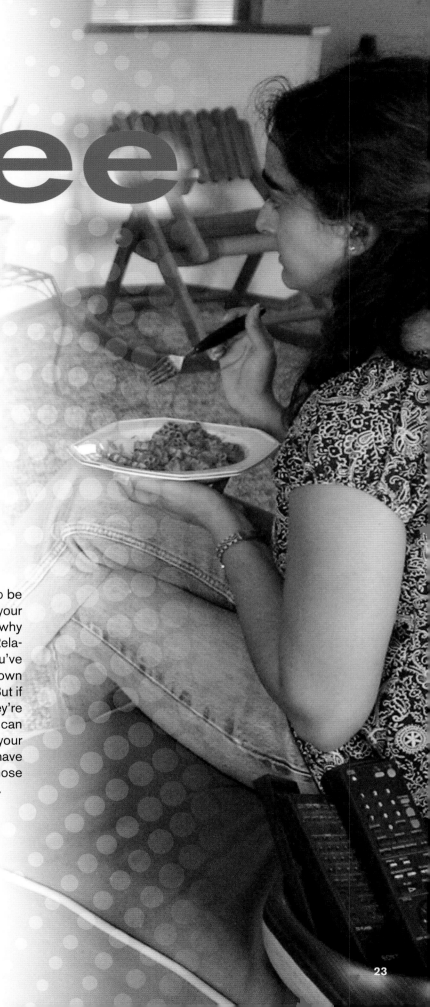

Chapter
Three

Overcoming
Challenges

In This Chapter

- Looking beyond the usual excuses
- Identifying the challenges you face
- Reviewing the benefits of an active life
- Practicing the art of problem solving

Health experts point to plenty of good reasons to be physically active, and you probably have a few on your list. You also probably have plenty of reasons for why it's hard to follow through. You're busy at work. Relatives are visiting. The holidays are coming up. You've hit a rough patch in your personal life and feel down in the dumps. All of these reasons may be valid. But if they're keeping you from achieving your goals, they're getting in the way of you being as healthy as you can be. This week, while you fit two-minute walks into your schedule, you'll ponder some of the reasons you have trouble finding time to be active. Recognizing those reasons is the first step to working around them.

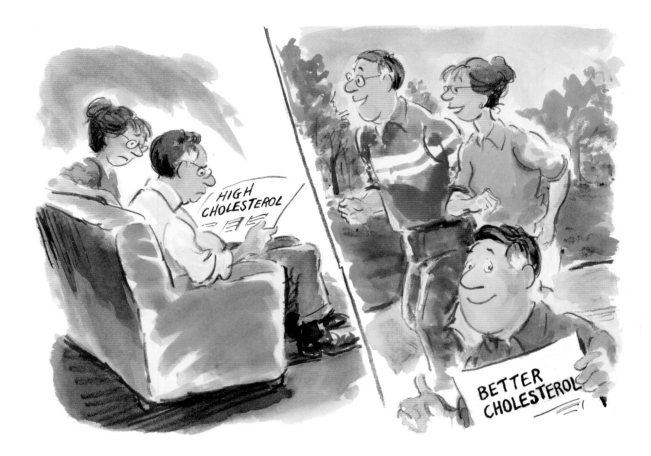

Excuses, Excuses

Why do the best-laid plans so often fall apart? Here are the three leading reasons we've heard from participants in our physical activity programs.

1. "I Just Don't Have the Time"

Nice try, but remember, we all have the same number of hours—168 to be exact—at our disposal each week. What varies is what we choose to do with them. Everyone has some leisure time to spend reading, watching TV, daydreaming, e-mailing, Twittering, or chatting on the phone. The question is this: Which of these activities can you cut back on to fit in additional physical activity each day? Are you willing to substitute some physical activity for something else you spend your time on now?

2. "I Don't Know How to Exercise"

Some people are sedentary because they think they don't know how to exercise properly. The only thing they lack is self-confidence. After all, you don't need any special skill to put one foot in front of another on a brisk walk. That's the appeal of adding simple, everyday activities to your life. You don't need special skills or fancy equipment. You don't have to know about target heart rates or special exercise approaches.

3. "I Can't Get the Help I Need"

We all have people around us who influence what we do and what we don't do. Those people play a key role when we're trying to make a change in our lives. Sometimes they can help, but unfortunately, sometimes they can hinder. If the people around you—your significant other, coworkers, or friends—aren't supportive, succeeding can be tough. Research has shown that having the support of friends and family members is especially important for adopting new physical activity habits. Later we'll give you some tips on how to get the support you need. For now, it's important to realize that being active is up to you. You can make it happen. To do that, however, you have to make it a top priority, and you have to make sure the people around you understand how much it matters.

Real Life

As a kid, George wasn't good at sports. Most of his life, in fact, he avoided exercise. In his 40s, George realized how important becoming physically active was to his health. Learning that his blood pressure and cholesterol levels were too high gave him a nudge. He joined a club and started lifting weights and jogging. After the second day, he was so sore he could hardly get out of bed. The bad experience confirmed his sense that exercise wasn't for him. Luckily, George didn't give up. In our program, he learned that there are many ways to be active. He came to understand that doing what you love is the best way to become active and stick with it. He also learned to take lifestyle changes one step at a time.

These days, George walks whenever he can. He takes stairs instead of elevators and escalators. He plans active things to do on weekends, such as hiking and riding a bicycle. He's lost a little weight and his cholesterol and blood pressure numbers have come down. More importantly, he has never felt better in his life. He knows that he is improving his health by being active.

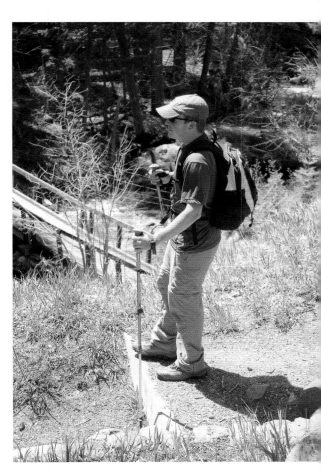

Myth Buster

"You can't tell me gardening counts as exercise."

True, sitting on your haunches and pulling weeds or planting seeds doesn't count. But raking leaves, mowing the grass with a push mower, or digging a new flower or vegetable bed are all moderate- to vigorous-intensity activities, depending on how hard you go at them. Most people can tell if they're just puttering in the garden or really working hard. If you're working hard at what you do, gardening counts as exercise.

Meeting the Challenges You Face

For the participants in our study, obstacles to being active came in all shapes and sizes. One woman had to care for her elderly mother, which left her too tired to do activities for herself. One man just couldn't find the motivation to be active even though he loved watching sports.

Each of these people found ways around their particular problems. The woman taking care of her mother arranged for other family members to provide care for two afternoons a week. She fit in physical activity on those days and early in the morning before her mother woke up. The increased activity soon helped her feel less tired and less isolated.

The man who loved to follow sports realized that he didn't have to be a serious athlete to be active. Since he enjoyed going to the local playing field on Saturdays to watch softball games, he began going half an hour early and walking briskly around the field before the game. During breaks in the action he took a lap or two around the field. It didn't take long before he began to think of himself as an active person. With his newfound interest in being active, his wife bought him the *Wii Fit* video game for a birthday present. Now, instead of passively watching tennis or golf on television, he participates in a game or two of his own.

 ## Activity Alert

Identifying Your Challenges

 As you go through the week, be conscious of anything that seems to get in the way of your plan. Make a list of those challenges. As you might guess, we'll ask you about them later. You can also download a copy of this form from the ALED Online Web site.

My Challenges

1. _____
2. _____
3. _____
4. _____
5. _____
6. _____
7. _____
8. _____

From S.N. Blair, A.L. Dunn, B.H. Marcus, R.A. Carpenter, and P. Jaret, 2011, *Active Living Every Day*, 2nd ed. (Champaign, IL: Human Kinetics).

 ## Activity Alert

Identifying Benefits of Physical Activity

One way to motivate yourself is to remember the important benefits that physical activity can provide. All of us have one or two things that are especially important to us. They represent benefits that are powerful enough to get us going even when we're not in the mood. Benefits that our participants often listed included feeling productive, enjoying improved communication with a spouse, and feeling good about their bodies. It's important to identify the benefits that matter to *you*. Take a few minutes now to list the most important benefits you can gain by exercising. Again, as you go through your week, keep adding to your list.

You can also download a copy of this form from the ALED Online Web site.

My Benefits From Physical Activity

1. _____
2. _____
3. _____
4. _____
5. _____
6. _____
7. _____
8. _____

From S.N. Blair, A.L. Dunn, B.H. Marcus, R.A. Carpenter, and P. Jaret, 2011, *Active Living Every Day*, 2nd ed. (Champaign, IL: Human Kinetics).

An Encouraging Word

The evidence from scientific studies is as solid as a rock: Physical activity is crucial to good health and overall well-being. Here's what we know for certain.

- People who are physically active are less likely than people who are inactive to develop heart disease and some types of cancer, such as colon cancer, lung cancer, and breast cancer.
- As they get older, active people have a better quality of life, suffer fewer disabilities, and are more likely to remain independent than inactive people.
- Physical activity helps keep blood pressure down, minimizes bone loss with age, and substantially lowers the risk of developing type 2 diabetes.
- Physical activity helps people maintain their weight effectively.
- People who are regularly active report feeling less stressed and more able to cope with life than when they were inactive. Studies also suggest that active people are less likely to feel depressed or anxious than sedentary people.
- Many people report feeling more energetic and productive than before they increased their activity.
- People who become physically active often report sleeping better than when they were inactive.

You've given some thought to the reasons why you aren't as active as you'd like to be. Now take a moment to remind yourself of the benefits of being active. Long-term benefits such as lower risk of heart disease and other chronic illnesses are important, of course. But if these seem too far away to offer much motivation, remember that there are also quick rewards to getting up and moving, such as an improved outlook or increased energy.

The Art of Problem Solving

You've already identified your personal challenges. The next step is to use some simple problem-solving skills. Problem solving simply means thinking creatively about the most effective solution when a problem—or an obstacle—blocks your way. Behavioral scientists have devised many problem-solving models.

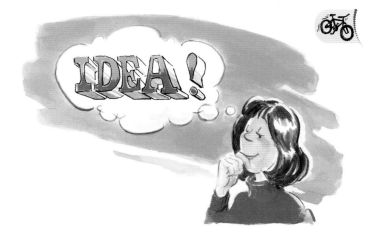

🚲 Activity Alert

Think IDEA

Here's a simple approach that seemed to work well for participants in our program. Just think IDEA: Identify the problem, develop a list of solutions, evaluate the solutions, and analyze how well the plan worked.

Identify the Problem

Remember that list of challenges? From the list you made, choose one. Write it down in the first section of the Great IDEA! form on the next page. Take a moment to think about the specifics. What in particular keeps you from being active? Perhaps you are having trouble being active on your many business trips. Travel may make you feel too tired to be physically active, or perhaps you don't feel safe or comfortable walking or doing other activities in an unfamiliar place. Maybe you're working a second job to make ends meet, and you just don't have much free time to walk or ride a bike. Or maybe you're facing tough times and finding it hard to get motivated. Write down the most important details about your personal barrier.

Develop a List of Solutions

Be creative. Don't worry whether the solutions are good or bad, workable or unrealistic; that will come later. Sometimes your wildest idea will turn out to be the best solution. Jot down all the ideas you can come up with. Keep your list with you over the next few days, and add any other solutions that come to mind.

Evaluate Your Solutions

Select one of the ideas you've written down that you're willing to try. Then develop a specific plan for how and when you can put it to the test. Here's what a plan might look like. Let's say your downfall is business trips. The problem is that you don't feel comfortable walking in an unfamiliar area. One plan might involve checking ahead to make sure your hotel has an exercise facility. Another solution might involve learning a set of simple aerobic exercises you can do in the comfort of your hotel room. A third strategy might be walking as much as you can instead of sitting at the airport. It should be easy to get motivated. After all, there is no better way to fully experience a new city than to get out and walk or run. Be sure to ask the hotel desk clerk about safe places and times to go. Hotel staff members are usually more than happy to tell you about the most interesting places in the area.

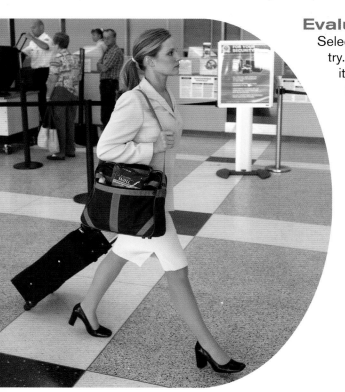

Even if you travel a lot, you can find ways to be active at the airport or the hotel.

Analyze How Well Your Plan Worked

After you have given your plan a try, analyze how well it worked. Be honest. This is the time to revise your plan before you try again. Maybe all it needs is a little tinkering, or maybe it needs more revising than that. If your plan fell flat on its face, come up with another by starting at the beginning of the IDEA process.

 Use the Great IDEA! form whenever you have a problem you need to solve. Photocopy the form in this book so you have plenty on hand, or download it from the ALED Online Web site.

Great IDEA!

I–Identify a barrier that keeps you from being active.

_____

_____

_____

D–Develop a few creative solutions (the more the merrier).

_____

_____

_____

E–Evaluate your list of solutions. In the following space, write the solution you are willing to try. Write down precisely when and how you will put it into action.

_____

_____

_____

A–Analyze how well your plan worked and revise it if necessary. If your plan worked well, give it five stars. If it only deserves two stars, write down how it could become a five-star plan. If your plan bombed completely, look back at your list of solutions and try again. (Remember, a plan that doesn't work isn't a complete failure. It often points toward the solution that *will* work. The only failure is giving up).

_____

_____

_____

From S.N. Blair, A.L. Dunn, B.H. Marcus, R.A. Carpenter, and P. Jaret, 2011, *Active Living Every Day*, 2nd ed. (Champaign, IL: Human Kinetics).

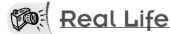 **Real Life**

Ida had plenty of reasons to increase her activity. She was overweight, her blood pressure was too high, and heart disease ran in her family. With three teenagers at home and a job as an office manager for a large construction company, however, she never seemed to find the time to exercise. On top of that, her husband seemed threatened by the idea that she wanted to be more active.

Ida began by listing all the things that kept her from being active. Then she started developing solutions. Within 20 minutes she had about 20 ideas—some reasonable, some zany. Here's part of her list:

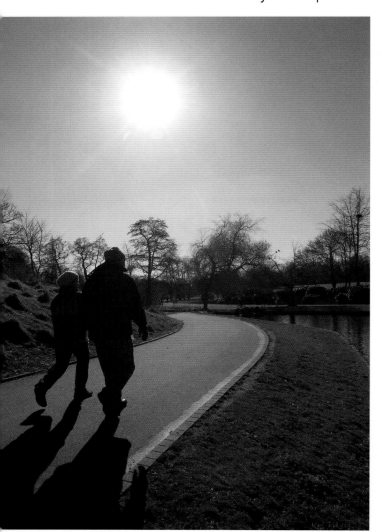

- Walking around while using the phone to order building materials
- Taking a 10-minute walk during lunch and break time
- Talking to her husband about her interest in being more active and encouraging him to join in
- Taking a talk-and-walk with her husband two nights a week instead of just turning on the television
- Walking around the baseball field during the kids' games
- Walking to the corner grocery store instead of driving
- Asking the kids to take over a few household chores (with a little extra allowance thrown in) to create extra time for a brisk walk through the neighborhood after dinner

Ida decided to talk to her husband about her commitment to being more active. She also decided to ask him to walk with her for half an hour instead of watching television. Finally, she committed to taking a 10-minute walk over the lunch hour. Her husband proved to be very supportive. He and Ida agreed to think of their evening walk as a date. They talked about the kids, their work, and what was going on in the neighborhood. Before long they went from two nights a week to three. Ida was so encouraged by the success of her first plan that she went back to her list of solutions and selected another: walking around the baseball field during the kids' games.

 Myth Buster

"I've tried and failed so many times, I'm beginning to think I'm not cut out for exercise."

There are two myths at work here. First is the idea that slipping now and then means you've failed. No one succeeds without a few slips along the way. Slips can even be helpful by spotlighting obstacles or showing where your plan needs tinkering. The second myth is that some people aren't cut out for exercise. Exercise is just a fancy word for physical activity, after all. Our bodies were designed to be physically active. Anthropologists believe that early hunter-gatherers walked or ran up to 20 miles (32 km) a day just to socialize. We can't live the way they did, nor would we want to. But all of us have some kind of physical activity we can enjoy and feel good about.

Moving Forward

Health experts now know that being inactive is a big problem for many people. It can rob you of health, energy, and even happiness. Luckily, as with most problems, you can solve inactivity with a little ingenuity and persistence. This week, you've identified one of your biggest challenges and developed some solutions. You've evaluated those solutions, analyzing what does and doesn't work for you. No matter what problem you face, these steps offer a useful way to understand what you're up against and find ways around it. If you're stuck in a rut, look back at the last two weeks to find ways to encourage and motivate yourself.

CHAPTER CHECKLIST

Before you move on to the next week's activities, make sure you've done the following:

- Identified obstacles that prevent you from being active
- Listed at least three important benefits of increasing your activity
- Filled out the Great IDEA! form

 Checked out chapter 3 on the ALED Online Web site for more helpful resources and information for this chapter

Chapter Four

Setting Goals and Rewarding Yourself

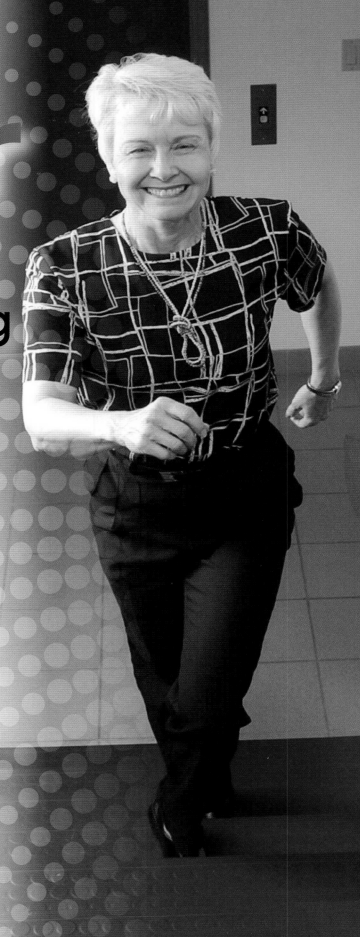

In This Chapter

- Setting goals
- Identifying rewards that will keep you motivated
- Taking the stairs
- Writing down positive messages

In a famous exchange from Lewis Carroll's *Alice's Adventures in Wonderland*, Alice asked the Cheshire Cat this question:

"Would you tell me, please, which way I ought to walk from here?"

"That depends a good deal on where you want to get to," said the Cat.

"I don't much care where," said Alice.

"Then it doesn't matter which way you walk," said the Cat.

The point is simple: You must have a destination in mind in order to know how to get there. That's especially true when you're trying to change something important in your life. We know from our own research that setting goals is one of the keys to success. The clearer your goal, the better your odds of reaching it.

Measuring Success

To set and achieve a goal, you need a way to measure your progress. There are several ways to measure physical activity. You can add up the time you spend doing an activity such as walking. As an alternative, you can use the Energy Expenditure Chart in appendix C, pages 161-164, to add up how many calories you burn. A little later in this book we'll show you another useful way to measure physical activity: using a step counter to set a daily physical activity goal.

Measuring your progress is important for many reasons. It can help keep you motivated. It can help you pace yourself. It also lets you know when you've reached milestones along the way to meeting your goal.

Tips for Goal Setting

It's not enough simply to say, "I want to become more active." Learning how to set a specific, measurable goal is crucial to success. Here are four important tips that should help.

1. Be as specific as you can.

People who set specific goals do better than people who say, "I'll try to do my best." For example, instead of saying, "This week I'll try to get more exercise," set a specific goal of walking for 15 minutes at every lunch hour during the week and another 15 minutes after dinner on five nights of the week.

2. Make it personal.

Your goals should be ones that *you* believe in and want to attain, not something someone else said you should do. You are more likely to stay focused if you set a goal that matters to you.

3. Be realistic.

Consider your current physical activity and fitness level. If you are just getting started, set a goal that is a bit challenging but still doable. Drastic changes are hard to accomplish and even harder to maintain. Often it is best to break a big goal into several smaller, more realistic goals.

4. Give yourself feedback.

Choose a way to track your progress. You may want to add up the time you spend walking or performing other activities. Or, you may want to use the Energy Expenditure Chart to tally up calories (see pages 161-164 in appendix C). Track your progress day by day and week by week. There will be times when you exceed your goals, and there will also be times when you fall behind. By monitoring your progress, you'll begin to see the pattern of ups and downs and understand that the downs are only temporary.

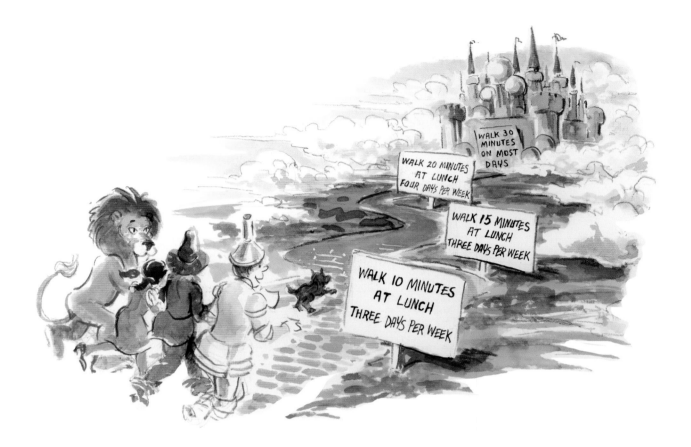

Set Short-Term and Long-Term Goals

A journey of a thousand miles begins with the first step, as the Chinese proverb says. Short-term goals, in other words, are important if you want to go the distance. If your long-term goal is to walk an hour a day, five days a week, don't expect to reach that goal all at once. A good short-term goal might be to walk for two 15-minute bouts on Saturday, Tuesday, and Thursday. Then gradually increase the number of minutes and the number of days per week that you walk. Short-term goals can be as brief as one day or several weeks. You can set your long-term goals for a month or two in the future.

 ## Activity Alert

Ready? Set? Goals!

Using the form on page 36, set a goal you intend to meet. Remember to be as specific as you can. For instance, if your activity is walking, specify how many minutes you plan to walk and when you will do it. Be explicit about how you will monitor your progress. Decide how far into the future your long-term goal should be. Some people set a one-month goal. Others prefer a longer goal, such as two months. Be careful not to set a goal so big or so far off that you lose sight of it and get discouraged. You can also download a copy of this form from the ALED Online Web site.

My Goals

A long-term goal I plan to achieve by _____ (date) is

_____

_____

_____

How I plan to monitor my progress

_____

_____

_____

Short-term goals that will help me reach my long-term goal

1. _____

2. _____

3. _____

1. How I plan to monitor my progress

_____

_____

_____

2. How I plan to monitor my progress

_____

_____

_____

3. How I plan to monitor my progress

_____

_____

_____

_____

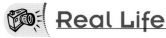

Real Life

Carlos was like many high school athletes. He tried to stay active after he started a career and family. Before long, however, he found himself watching more sports than he played. Once or twice a year he'd run, but it was painful and discouraging. Then Carlos saw an ad on television about Project *Active*, and he decided to join. He learned about two-minute walks and began adding them to his day. Once he got the hang of two-minute walks, he began planning his day to include several 10-minute walks. Instead of his usual fast-food lunch, he brought a bag lunch and took a 20-minute walk.

Eventually he set a goal of walking and running in his neighborhood three nights a week. Before long, his goal became more focused. He challenged himself to run a 10K race. Then he set a goal of playing in a charity basketball event.

Both of these long-term goals helped motivate Carlos to get back in shape. To meet them, he divided them into specific short-term goals. During his evening walks and runs, for instance, he would try to add one block each week. Sure, he had some setbacks along the way. But he managed to make physical activity a regular part of his life again.

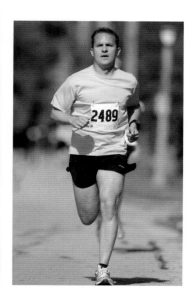

Value of Rewards

Knowing the benefits of an active life can help motivate you. But we've also learned from our work how important small rewards can be, especially when they are tied to attaining goals. Anyone who has ever trained a puppy knows how important treats are to changing behavior. People are no different. We reach further and achieve more when we know there's a reward (though not necessarily food treats) waiting for us at the end of the line. The feeling of satisfaction after finishing a race may be its own reward. But let's face it—it's also nice to get that T-shirt at the finish line.

In most things you set out to do, there's an intrinsic reward that comes from feeling confident and in control. That's important. In fact, psychologists have developed the field of self-determination theory to describe the effect of such intrinsic rewards. Despite its fancy name, the notion is fairly simple. We all have a need to feel competent at something. That feeling of competence offers its own reward when we do something like take on a new activity. In addition, all of us need to feel related to other people. Any activity that gives us that feeling also has its own rewards. We all want to have a sense of autonomy—of being the masters of our own fate. Again, any activity that gives us that sense offers its own intrinsic reward.

Being physically active fulfills many of these basic needs. It offers a way to feel competent, to connect to others, and to control your health and well-being. Many people are active simply because it feels good on so many levels. They like to feel in control, they enjoy walking or cycling or going to a spinning class with others, and they like to feel competent at what they do. By now, you may have experienced some of these intrinsic rewards. If so, they'll help to keep you motivated.

Sometimes it helps to plan an extrinsic reward, too. By that we mean something tangible, such as a special book, theater tickets, a fancy dinner, or even a vacation. Rewards can help focus your efforts and boost your motivation. Rewards are especially important to help get you through the rough patches when you're feeling discouraged or frustrated.

Real Life

Louis was doing fine, working out regularly and keeping his weight and cholesterol down. Then his company transferred him to a new location. Suddenly he couldn't find time to get to the gym. Within a few months, his cholesterol was up and his waistline was expanding.

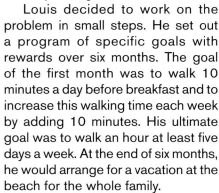

Louis decided to work on the problem in small steps. He set out a program of specific goals with rewards over six months. The goal of the first month was to walk 10 minutes a day before breakfast and to increase this walking time each week by adding 10 minutes. His ultimate goal was to walk an hour at least five days a week. At the end of six months, he would arrange for a vacation at the beach for the whole family.

Louis told his wife and family about his goal and the reward he'd promised himself when he reached it. His wife began to call him at work just before lunchtime to encourage him. At home his kids cheered him on. He and his wife decided that they would try something on their vacation that they'd always wanted to do—scuba diving. As they planned the trip, Louis got increasingly motivated to reach his goal. He wanted to have enough energy to enjoy diving. Most of all, he wanted to make sure he earned the reward of a special vacation. By the fourth month, he and his wife were both walking half an hour in the morning or in the evening. Louis had added another 30 minutes by taking 10-minute walks throughout the day.

Did You Know?

Researchers are exploring a novel way to motivate change for the better: betting money on it. In one example, people who hope to lose weight get together and bet against one another to see who can lose the most weight. In another, a team of people who want to become more active bet on who will tally up the most minutes of activity each week. In some cases the bet is between friends, such as one person betting the other that she will quit smoking once and for all.

The bets are typically for small amounts, but money isn't really the point. Making a bet with someone to accomplish your goal can offer a powerful incentive. A study at the Philadelphia Veterans Affairs Medical Center found that dieters with an economic incentive were far more successful at shedding weight than those who were motivated simply to lose weight. After 16 weeks, a control group lost just under 4 pounds (1.8 kg). The two groups with monetary incentives lost 13 to 14 pounds (5.9-6.3 kg). About half of those with money at stake met their 16-week goal, compared with only about 10 percent of those with no financial incentive. Keep in mind that this strategy works best as a short-term motivator. Dieters have to use other ways to stick with their commitment to maintaining a healthy weight. Still, economic incentives seem to be powerful motivators (Volpp et al. 2008).

You can use this strategy to make any change. For instance, a group of people at an insurance company got together to become more active by walking during lunch and breaks. They each contributed a dollar a week. At the end of three months, the person who tallied up the most active time won the money.

Creative Rewards

You would think rewarding ourselves would be easy, but often it's not. We're used to congratulating and encouraging our loved ones. Most of the time, though, we don't bother to congratulate ourselves.

Stumped for ideas on how to reward yourself? Here are a few of the special treats that worked well for Project *Active* participants:

Massages	New pair of comfortable work shoes
New walking or running shoes	Biking vacation
Theater or sport tickets	Manicure or facial
Bottle of wine	Night at a bed-and-breakfast
New hairdo	Fresh flowers
New bracelet	Small piece of chocolate
New watch	Visit with friends
Bubble bath	Trip to a local museum
New workout clothes	Movie
New MP3 player	Dinner at a favorite restaurant
Dance class	New album or song download
Night out for dancing	New bike
New magazine or newsletter sub-scription	New walking shoes
	New blouse or shirt
Flying a kite with friends or family	Alone time for yourself

Did You Know?

In Project *Active* and in our studies at Brown University, we measured the strategies that people use to meet their goals. People who use rewards, we discovered, are far more likely to remain active over time than those who don't.

Activity Alert

Identifying Rewards

It's time to reward yourself for all the good work you're doing or plan to do. Think about your specific goals, both short and long term. Look back at the form you filled in on page 36. Now list a few ways you can reward yourself for achieving your short-term goals. If your goal is to lose weight, of course, an ice cream sundae may not be the best reward. Choose a reward that helps you move toward your goal, not away from it! You can also download a copy of the form on page 40 from the ALED Online Web site.

Small Rewards for Short-Term Goals

_____
_____
_____
_____
_____
_____

 Now think big. Write down ideas for rewards that might help spur you on toward your long-term goal. You can also download a copy of this form from the ALED Online Web site.

Big Rewards for Long-Term Goals

_____
_____
_____
_____
_____

Go back to the long-term and short-term goals that you set on page 36. Choose a reward that you'll give yourself for reaching each goal.

Once you've put your commitment in writing, chances are you'll take it seriously. If you want some added insurance, have a friend or family member sign as a witness to your goals and rewards. It may sound silly at first, but studies show that peer pressure can go a long way toward motivating us when the going gets tough!

Step Right Up

By now you've discovered a variety of ways to add brisk walks to your daily routine. Climbing stairs is one that many people overlook. It's an option many of us can take advantage of at work, the mall, the airport or bus terminal, and other places we go. Most of us never give it a second thought. Instead of taking the stairs, we take the elevator or escalator. No wonder—in places such as shopping malls, it's often hard to even find the staircase. Whereas the escalators are right in the middle of the building, surrounded by beautiful displays of flowers or merchandise, the staircase is usually in a dim corner.

Don't let that discourage you. Climbing stairs burns almost 10 times more calories than riding up the elevator or escalator. Stair-climbing burns two to three times as many calories as walking because with each step up, you lift your body weight (plus whatever you're carrying). Climbing stairs burns as many calories per minute as jogging, playing racquetball or tennis, or hiking with a heavy backpack. And you'll give your leg and buttock muscles a little tune-up—not bad for a few flights of stairs.

Activity Alert

Taking the Stairs

Take a moment to think about where you go and what you do during the day. Are there opportunities to take the stairs instead of an escalator or elevator? Is there a staircase you can climb when you take a break at work? Make a list of opportunities for stair-climbing in your daily life.

Stair-Climbing Opportunities

1. _____
2. _____
3. _____
4. _____
5. _____

From S.N. Blair, A.L. Dunn, B.H. Marcus, R.A. Carpenter, and P. Jaret, 2011, *Active Living Every Day*, 2nd ed. (Champaign, IL: Human Kinetics).

 ## Did You Know?

Researchers at the University of Ulster and Queen's University Belfast conducted a study with 15 inactive young women who were divided into two groups (Boreham et al. 2005). The women in one group maintained their usual activities, while those in the other group added stair-climbing every day. Each day during the first week, they climbed a single, long staircase with 199 steps, which took approximately 135 seconds. The second week, they climbed two flights of stairs over the course of each day. By the end of seven weeks, they were climbing six flights of stairs, not all at once but with an hour or so between climbs. Compared with the inactive women, the stair-climbers increased their fitness, lowered their total cholesterol levels, and improved their ratio of good to bad cholesterol! That's a big payoff for less than 14 minutes of stair-climbing each day.

 ## Real Life

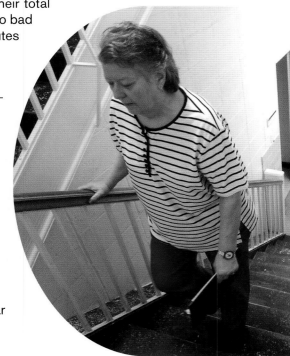

Elena traveled frequently to Central and South America in her work as a buyer for a leading import company. When she was home, she managed to stick to her activity plan. But when she was on the road, she often found it difficult to be active.

One day a colleague told her that he'd had the same problem until he realized that stairwells in hotels were a perfect way to get a quick workout almost anywhere. The next time Elena traveled, she asked the hotel manager for a room on the fourth floor. In the morning, in the late afternoon, and again in the evening, she climbed up and down the stairs twice. In the end, she made stair-climbing a regular part of her travel plans.

? Did You Know?

Researchers at the University of Pennsylvania devised a clever physical activity experiment (Brownell, Stunkard, and Albaum 1980). Observing a public transit station for a few days, they counted how many people took the escalator versus the stairs. Not surprisingly, many more people opted for the easy way up rather than the climb. Then the researchers posted a sign telling people to take the stairs for a healthy heart. Immediately, many more people began taking the stairs. When the sign was posted, stair use doubled compared with the baseline. When the researchers then removed their sign, stair use steadily declined. Within a few months, the commuters were back to their old habit of riding the escalator.

The bottom line is that we'd all improve our health if we had ways to remind ourselves about the many opportunities we have to be physically active. Here's another strategy: Keep track of every flight of stairs you climb (for example, carry a small notebook in your purse or a piece of folded paper in your wallet, and add a check mark each time you climb a flight). Set a goal for climbing 25 flights. When you reach your goal, reward yourself. Then set a new, even more ambitious goal.

Zen of Activity

One important reward of an active lifestyle is improved health and increased energy. We hope you're already beginning to feel a little fitter now than before you increased your activity. If you have energy to spare when you need it to run for the bus or climb a steep set of stairs, you're already experiencing the intrinsic benefits of activity.

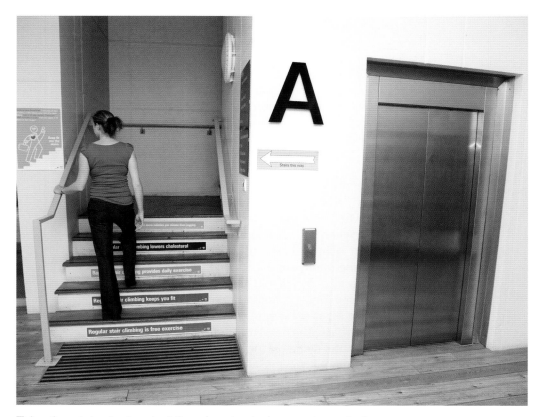

Take the stairs instead of the elevator to burn extra calories.

Take time this week to become more aware of the here-and-now pleasures of physical activity. Moving, feeling your heart kick up, seeing the world around you, improving your self-confidence, learning a new skill—all of these are important pleasures. They are the intrinsic rewards we talked about earlier. Next time you engage in physical activity, take a few minutes to savor the experience. Enjoy the sights, sounds, and smells you encounter along the way. Feel your arms and legs moving. Be aware of your heart beating. After you're through with the activity, take in a deep breath and let it out slowly.

It feels great to be active.

Activity Alert

Pat Yourself on the Back

The messages we give ourselves can have a big impact on what we achieve. If the messages are negative, such as "I'm no good at sticking with a plan" or "I'm always too tired at the end of the day to do anything," it's easy to get discouraged. However, if you encourage yourself with positive messages, such as "All I need is 10 minutes to relax, then I'm ready for anything" or "I can do anything if I put my heart into it," you're likely to succeed.

Take a few minutes now to think of some positive things to say to yourself about being physically active. Some examples might include the following:

- "It may be hard for me to get going sometimes, but once I get over that first hurdle, there's no stopping me."
- "Just getting up and moving makes me feel better."
- "I've solved bigger problems. I can figure out where to find another 10 minutes for activity."

Write down at least two messages on page 44 that will inspire and encourage you. You may also want to write them on a piece of paper you keep in your wallet for those moments when you need a little push.

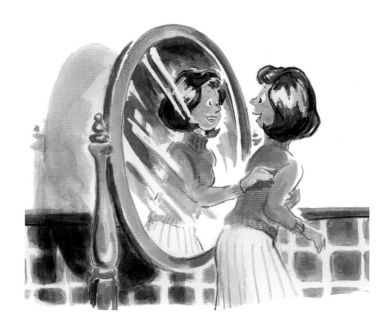

Messages to Inspire Me

1. _____
2. _____
3. _____
4. _____
5. _____

From S.N. Blair, A.L. Dunn, B.H. Marcus, R.A. Carpenter, and P. Jaret, 2011, *Active Living Every Day*, 2nd ed. (Champaign, IL: Human Kinetics).

 # Real Life

Mariel had gone through a tough year. She'd lost her job as a receptionist when the downturn hit, and it took her almost two months to find another job. A single mom with two small kids, she had to watch every penny. With the stress of being unemployed, she stopped going out for walks and began eating junk food. Within a month she had gained 6 pounds (2.7 kg). Worse than that, she began to think of herself as a failure in almost everything she did.

Luckily, she knew that wasn't really true. To counter the negative message, she wrote a list of the things she was proud of accomplishing. Her list included, "No matter how tired I feel, I can always find energy to play with the kids," and "Once I set a goal, I can reach it."

She immediately set a goal to take three 10-minute walks each day for the rest of the week. She also made plans to take the kids to the playground after school, where they could all be active together. When she finally found another job, she rewarded herself and the kids with a day at a local amusement park.

Having a specific goal and reward will focus your commitment and help you through the rough patches. Along the way, it's important to talk positively to yourself. It will help you stay motivated to achieve your goals.

CHAPTER CHECKLIST

Before you move on to the next week's activities, make sure you've done the following:

- Listed your short-term and long-term physical activity goals
- Identified rewards for attaining your short-term and long-term goals
- Made plans to monitor your progress
- Identified at least one opportunity to climb stairs during the day
- Made a list of positive messages to encourage yourself

 Checked out chapter 4 on the ALED Online Web site for more helpful resources and information for this chapter

References

Boreham et al. 2005. Training effects of short bouts of stair climbing on cardiorespiratory fitness, blood lipids, and homocysteine in sedentary young women. *British Journal of Sports Medicine* 39(9): 590-593.

Brownell, K.D., A.J. Stunkard, and J.M. Albaum. 1980. Evaluation and modification of exercise patterns in the natural environment. *American Journal of Psychiatry* 137(12): 1540-1545.

Volpp et al. 2008. Financial incentive-based approaches for weight loss: a randomized trial. *Journal of the American Medical Association* 300(22): 2631-2637.

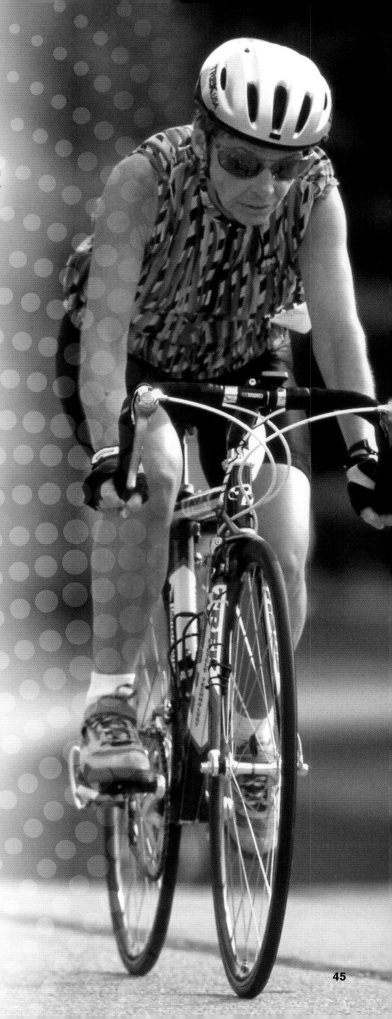

Chapter Five

Gaining Confidence

In This Chapter

- Understanding energy expenditure in physical activity
- Identifying light-, moderate-, and vigorous-intensity activities
- Finding ways to burn an extra 1,000 calories per week
- Tallying minutes spent in moderate- or vigorous-intensity activities
- Replacing negative messages with positive messages
- Turning errands into opportunities for activity

To reach a goal, you need to start with a plan. Just as important, you have to know how to measure your progress. Over the past weeks you've been adding up the amount of time you spend every day doing some kind of physical activity. You've learned that you can substitute active time for sedentary time. You've discovered that accumulating small bits of physical activity can add up to big health benefits.

This week, you'll try out another way of measuring progress—calculating how much energy (measured as calories) you burn being physically active. Why bother? Because research shows that whether you do your activity in short bouts or long bouts, at moderate intensity or vigorous intensity, the goal is to increase the total amount of calories you burn being physically active over a day, week, or month.

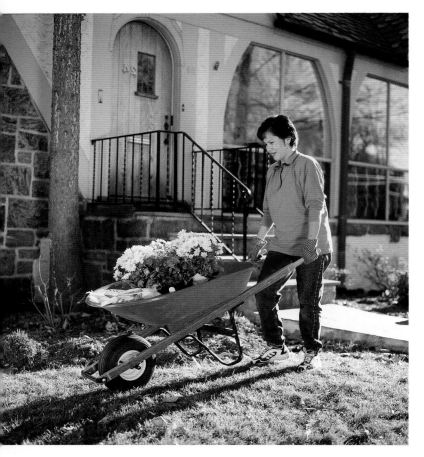

Regardless of the activity you choose and how often you do it, what matters is how much energy you expend over a day, week, or month.

Measuring energy expenditure isn't rocket science. It does require a little math, however. Energy expenditure depends on four things:

- Your current body weight
- How hard you push yourself (intensity)
- How much time you spend engaging in an activity (duration)
- How often you do the activity (frequency)

Together, these factors determine how many calories you burn when you're physically active. Let's take a closer look.

Body Size Does Matter

A 200-pound (90.7 kg) person is going to burn more calories than a 140-pound (63.5 kg) person doing the same activity. Why? A larger body has more mass to move around. Imagine taking a walk around the block or up a couple flights of stairs. Then imagine doing the same thing loaded down with a 20-pound (9.1 kg) bag of sand. The walk would feel much harder. Along the way, you would also burn more calories.

How many extra calories? Compare Flora, who weighs only 140 pounds (63.5 kg), with Tom, who tips the scale at 200 pounds (90.7 kg):

	Estimated calories burned per min	
	Flora **140 lb (63.5 kg)**	**Tom** **200 lb (90.7 kg)**
Walking at moderate pace **20 min per mi (1.6 km)**	3.7	5.3

Walking at the same speed, Tom burns more calories per minute than Flora. This is because his heart, lungs, and muscles work harder than Flora's to move his bigger body.

A Closer Look at Intensity

Next, let's look at exercise intensity. The more vigorous the activity, the more energy (calories) you burn each minute. Again, compare Flora and Tom as they do various activities.

Physical activity	Intensity category	Estimated calories burned per min	
		Flora 140 lb (63.5 kg)	Tom 200 lb (90.7 kg)
Walking			
30 min per mi (1.6 km) pace	Light	2.8	4.0
20 min per mi pace	Moderate	3.7	5.3
15 min per mi pace	Moderate	5.6	8.0
12 min per mi pace	Vigorous	9.0	12.7
Mowing lawn			
Riding mower	Light	2.8	4.0
Power mower, walk behind	Moderate	5.0	7.2
Hand mower, no power	Vigorous	6.7	9.6

This table shows how two common activities, walking and lawn mowing, can burn different numbers of calories depending on the intensity of the activity. You can see the difference in Flora's and Tom's energy expenditures.

We typically divide intensity into light, moderate, and vigorous. Light activities are those that burn 1 to 3 times the energy per minute as the body does at complete rest. Moderate activities burn 3 to 5.9 times the energy per minute, and vigorous activities burn 6 or more times the energy per minute. Here are some common activities at these levels of intensity:

Light

Working at a desk

Standing

Cooking

Chopping vegetables

Driving a car, dusting, watching TV, or reading

Moderate

Brisk walking

Raking

Weeding

Mopping

Sweeping

Vacuuming

Light weightlifting

Doing calisthenics

Golfing (no cart)

Biking at a slow pace (10 mi [16 km] per hour)

Swimming laps (less than 50 yd [45.7 m] per minute)

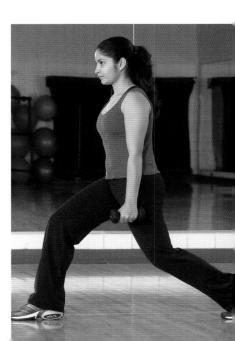

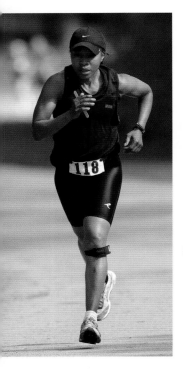

Vigorous

Stair-climbing

Scrubbing the floor

Digging in the garden

Doing heavy carpentry

Dancing (aerobic)

Playing tennis (singles)

Biking (13 mi [20.9 km] per hour or faster)

Playing soccer or basketball

Jumping rope

Running

Hiking in the mountains (going uphill)

Swimming laps (50-75 yd [45.7-68.6 m] per minute)

 ## Activity Alert

Checking Your Pace

One way to understand intensity is to pay attention to how physical activity feels as you're doing it. Try a simple experiment. Map out a .5-mile (.8 km) course in your neighborhood. (Your local high school may have a .25-mi [.4 km] track you can use.) One day this week, walk the course at your usual pace for .5 mile (.8 km). Keep track of your time using this page. Then use the time to determine the approximate intensity of your activity.

My time for the .5-mile (.8 km) circuit is _____.

Compare your time with the following chart. How are you doing?

Time	Intensity
More than 10 min	Light intensity
7.5 to 10 min	Moderate intensity
Less than 7.5 min	Vigorous intensity

From S.N. Blair, A.L. Dunn, B.H. Marcus, R.A. Carpenter, and P. Jaret, 2011, *Active Living Every Day*, 2nd ed. (Champaign, IL: Human Kinetics).

How Hard Do I Need to Push Myself?

Not long ago, exercise gurus made a big deal about exercise intensity. To get the benefits of exercise, they said, you needed to reach your target heart rate and stay there for at least 20 minutes. That required working up a serious sweat. OK, we'll admit it: We said the same thing ourselves. And we still think it's good advice for those who wish to do structured exercise and improve their fitness to a high level. However, most people simply need to move more. For most of us, regularly doing moderate-intensity activities such as walking briskly, playing golf, or working in the yard offers important health benefits.

The issue of intensity depends on who you are and what you want to achieve. Think for a moment about your starting place and your reasons for wanting to increase your activity. If, for instance, you're sedentary or unfit, then moderate-intensity activities will increase your fitness level and provide health benefits such as reduced blood pressure or cholesterol. What if you're already active and in good shape? You could do vigorous activities to improve your fitness and further reduce your health risks.

In It for the Duration

We've shown that body weight and exercise intensity are important to overall energy expenditure, as are the duration and frequency of physical activity. Let's go back to Flora and Tom. As the following table shows, the longer you do an activity, the more calories you burn.

	Estimated calories burned					
	Flora 140 lb (63.5 kg)			Tom 200 lb (90.7 kg)		
	Min			Min		
	10	30	60	10	30	60
Walking 30 min per mi 1.6 km) pace	28	94	168	44	132	264
20 min per mi pace	37	111	222	53	159	318
15 min per mi pace	56	168	336	80	240	480
12 min per mi pace	90	270	540	127	381	762

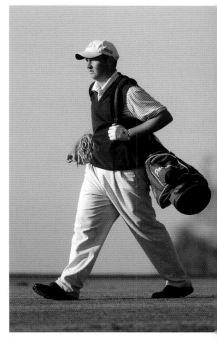

Even moderate-intensity activities such as walking the golf course offer important health benefits.

As you know by now, the goal is to do at least 150 minutes of moderate activity or 75 minutes of vigorous activity (or a combination of the two) each week. If you are physically active only a couple days a week rather than five days a week, you need to be active for longer durations each time in order to meet these goals. Or, you can break your daily goal into several 10-minute minisessions. Do whatever works best for you.

What's a good calorie goal to shoot for? That depends on your fitness level and your goal. Let's use Flora as an example. She wants to lose some weight, so she has decided to increase her daily amount of calories burned by being more active. She has set a goal to burn at least 1,000 extra calories each week. Here is how she plans to do it.

Physical activity	Calories per min *	Total time (min)	Total calories (calories per min × total time)
Walking, 20 min per mi (1.6 km)	3.7	120	444
Mowing lawn, power mower	5.0	30	150
Vacuuming vigorously	3.9	20	78
Bowling	3.4	40	136
Vigorous			
Playing tennis, doubles	6.7	40	268
Total weekly calories			**1, 076**

*For 140 lb (63.5 kg) person

(continued)

Monday	**Friday**
• Walk at lunch—15 min	• No activity
• Walk on break—15 min	**Saturday**
• Vacuum house—20 min	• Mow lawn—30 min
Tuesday	• Bowling—40 min
• Walk at lunch—30 min	**Sunday**
Wednesday	• Walk after lunch—45 min
• Tennis after work—40 min	
Thursday	
• Walk at lunch—15 min	

From S.N. Blair, A.L. Dunn, B.H. Marcus, R.A. Carpenter, and P. Jaret, 2011, *Active Living Every Day*, 2nd ed. (Champaign, IL: Human Kinetics).

As you can see, most of Flora's activities are at a moderate intensity. However, she plans to do a combination of activities to get her weekly extra 1,000 calories. That variety helps her to stay motivated and interested.

Did You Know?

In treating diabetes, a lot of attention is focused on a healthy diet. Diet is important, but we now know that physical activity and fitness are also vital for reducing risk. Studies from Harvard School of Public Health suggest that moderate and vigorous physical activity may prevent type 2 diabetes in many people (Hu et al. 1999). Activity can also protect people who are already diagnosed with this serious illness. In our studies, we found that men with diabetes who were unfit were twice as likely to die prematurely compared with fit men with diabetes. This was true even when we took into account other common risk factors such as high blood pressure, high blood cholesterol, smoking, obesity, family history of heart disease, and alcohol intake. We've long known that being physically active is important for otherwise healthy people. This study shows that people who have a difficult medical condition can also benefit from physical activity.

Activity Alert

Join the 1,000-Plus Club

People who want to lose weight often motivate themselves by thinking about how many calories they burn by being active. If you're among them, plan how you can burn at least 1,000 extra calories in a week. Note that at this stage in the ALED program, you may not be ready to burn 1,000 or more extra calories a week. Use the worksheet on page 51 as a guide for when you have built up your physical activity and fitness enough to do this amount of exercise.

- **Step 1.** Turn to pages 161-164. This chart shows per-minute calorie expenditure for activities at various body weights. Find the column that is closest to your weight.
- **Step 2.** Identify the moderate or vigorous activities you could do in one week to increase your physical activity. Be realistic! If you are sedentary, don't decide to run at a pace of eight minutes per mile (1.6 km) for 120 minutes. And don't forget those household chores and yard work that require at least moderate-intensity activity. They can add quite a few calories to your weekly total.
- **Step 3.** Once you have decided on the activities, play around with the amount of time you will spend in each activity.

Activity	Calories per min	Total time (min)	Total calories (calories per min × total time)
Moderate			
Vigorous			
	Total weekly calories		

From S.N. Blair, A.L. Dunn, B.H. Marcus, R.A. Carpenter, and P. Jaret, 2011, *Active Living Every Day*, 2nd ed. (Champaign, IL: Human Kinetics).

• **Step 4.** Plan how you will fit these activities into your week.

My Plan for Adding More Calorie-Burning Activities

Monday	
Tuesday	
Wednesday	
Thursday	
Friday	
Saturday	
Sunday	

 ## Real Life

No matter how often he reminded himself about the benefits of walking, Will still found it boring. He often felt it was a waste of time he'd rather use for something more worthwhile. Despite his best intentions, he frequently skipped his walk. Over time, he began to fall short of his goal to walk at least five nights a week after dinner.

Then for Christmas his wife gave him an MP3 player. He downloaded his favorite music. He popped on his headphones and listened the next time he went for a walk. He found himself so energized by the music that he walked an extra three blocks just to hear the end of the song. As a reward for meeting his goals each month—and to stay motivated—he treated himself to new song downloads. It was a great way to become physically active and build his music collection.

Activity Alert

Join the 150-Minute Club

If adding up calories is too much of a bother for you, here's an easier way to measure your progress. Just add up the amount of time you are active each day. Your goal will depend on who you are and how vigorously you exercise. Children and adolescents should do one hour or more of physical activity a day. That adds up to 420 minutes a week. If you have kids, that's a healthy goal to set for them. For adults aged 18 to 64, the 2008 Physical Activity Guidelines for Americans (Department of Health and Human Services 2008) call for at least

150 minutes of moderate per week, or

75 minutes of vigorous activities per week, or

a combination of moderate and vigorous activities.

By adding up even more active time, you can get even more health benefits. The ideal goal is to tally up 300 minutes of moderate activity or 150 minutes of vigorous activity each week. Don't be discouraged if you're not even close yet. Each step you take toward being more active is one step closer.

Weighing In

Burning More Calories Than You Eat

Each year hundreds of diet books hit the bookstores, each one claiming to offer the secret of dieting success. There is no secret, of course. The only way to lose weight is to burn more calories than you eat. You burn most calories in two ways: basic metabolism (energy used for breathing, body processes, and so on) and physical activity. You don't have much control over your metabolism. But you can change your activity level and eat a healthy diet.

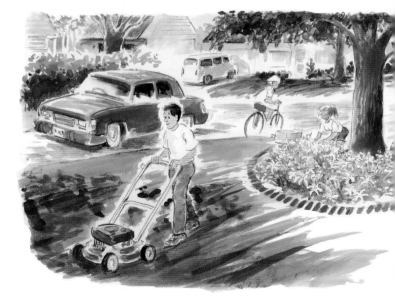

To lose 1 pound (.5 kg) in a week, you need to burn 3,500 more calories (about 500 calories per day) than you eat. This requires your body to call on its energy stores (body fat) to make up the energy deficit. You can do this by eating less, exercising more, or doing a combination of the two. Most people have trouble going hungry, which is what diets usually ask you to do. Being more active is easier for many people.

As you have seen, there are lots of ways to burn a little or a lot of extra calories. You can modify the intensity, duration, and frequency of your physical activities.

Keeping Track of Your Activities

By now we hope you're convinced that monitoring your activity in minutes or in calories can be a good way to find opportunities for activity and keep track of what you're doing. We have designed a handy self-monitoring form to help you keep track of the time you spend doing activities. And remember, if you haven't become active yet, you can still keep track of the times you think about doing activity on the Keeping Track of Thoughts form. Blank copies of the forms are located in appendix D on pages 166-167. Make copies of the forms you need and take them with you every day. You can also download a copy of this form from the ALED Online Web site. We guarantee that by monitoring your activity, you'll greatly increase your chances of success.

Keeping Track of Physical Activity

Instructions: This form is for you to check the amount of time you spend doing various activities. After doing an activity, mark the box that best describes the intensity of the activity (moderate or vigorous; see the Examples of Activities table on page 56) and its duration. At the end of the week, add the number of minutes checked for each activity category and place it in the column for total minutes.

Activity	Intensity level	2 min	10 min	Total min
Garden	Moderate	☐☐☐☐☐ ☐☐☐☐☐ ☐☐☐☐☐	☐☐☐☐☐ ☐☐☐☐☐ ☐☐☐☐☐	
	Vigorous	☐☐☐☐☐ ☐☐☐☐☐ ☐☐☐☐☐	☐☐☐☐☐ ☐☐☐☐☐ ☐☐☐☐☐	
Household	Moderate	☐☐☐☐☐ ☐☐☐☐☐ ☐☐☐☐☐	☐☐☐☐☐ ☐☐☐☐☐ ☐☐☐☐☐	
	Vigorous	☐☐☐☐☐ ☐☐☐☐☐ ☐☐☐☐☐	☐☐☐☐☐ ☐☐☐☐☐ ☐☐☐☐☐	
Leisure	Moderate	☐☐☐☐☐ ☐☐☐☐☐ ☐☐☐☐☐	☐☐☐☐☐ ☐☐☐☐☐ ☐☐☐☐☐	

Activity	Intensity level	2 min	10 min	Total min
	Vigorous	☐☐☐☐☐ ☐☐☐☐☐ ☐☐☐☐☐	☐☐☐☐☐ ☐☐☐☐☐ ☐☐☐☐☐	
Occupation	Moderate	☐☐☐☐☐ ☐☐☐☐☐ ☐☐☐☐☐	☐☐☐☐☐ ☐☐☐☐☐ ☐☐☐☐☐	
	Vigorous	☐☐☐☐☐ ☐☐☐☐☐ ☐☐☐☐☐	☐☐☐☐☐ ☐☐☐☐☐ ☐☐☐☐☐	
Sport	Moderate	☐☐☐☐☐ ☐☐☐☐☐ ☐☐☐☐☐	☐☐☐☐☐ ☐☐☐☐☐ ☐☐☐☐☐	
	Vigorous	☐☐☐☐☐ ☐☐☐☐☐ ☐☐☐☐☐	☐☐☐☐☐ ☐☐☐☐☐ ☐☐☐☐☐	
Stairs	Moderate (1 flight up = 10 steps)	☐☐☐☐☐ ☐☐☐☐☐ ☐☐☐☐☐	☐☐☐☐☐ ☐☐☐☐☐ ☐☐☐☐☐	
	Vigorous (4 flights up = 2 min vigorous work)	☐☐☐☐☐ ☐☐☐☐☐ ☐☐☐☐☐	☐☐☐☐☐ ☐☐☐☐☐ ☐☐☐☐☐	
Walking	Moderate	☐☐☐☐☐ ☐☐☐☐☐ ☐☐☐☐☐	☐☐☐☐☐ ☐☐☐☐☐ ☐☐☐☐☐	
	Vigorous	☐☐☐☐☐ ☐☐☐☐☐ ☐☐☐☐☐	☐☐☐☐☐ ☐☐☐☐☐ ☐☐☐☐☐	

From S.N. Blair, A.L. Dunn, B.H. Marcus, R.A. Carpenter, and P. Jaret, 2011, *Active Living Every Day*, 2nd ed. (Champaign, IL: Human Kinetics).

EXAMPLES OF ACTIVITIES

Activity	Moderate	Vigorous
Garden	Raking, mowing (push), weeding	Shoveling, carrying moderate or heavy loads
Household	Vacuuming carpet, cleaning windows	Moving furniture, shoveling snow
Leisure	Ballroom dancing, fishing from bank (standing or wading)	Pop dancing, backpacking
Occupation	Walking briskly at work	Using heavy tools, firefighting, loading or unloading truck, laying brick
Sport	Table tennis, golf (no cart), tai chi, Frisbee	Jumping rope, basketball, running, racquetball, soccer
Walking	15-20 min per mi (1.6 km) pace	Stair-climbing, mountain hiking

Did You Know?

By walking briskly for 10 minutes, you increase your breathing rate from 12 times to 35 times a minute. The amount of air in each breath increases fourfold, from about 1 pint (.47 L) to .5 gallon (1.9 L). All told, that means your body increases the volume of air you breathe twelvefold while you are walking fast. The result is a stronger heart and lungs and improved stamina.

Buying a Step Counter

Now we want to introduce you to one more handy way to track your activity—a step counter, or pedometer. We will go into more detail about how to use it in chapter 8. For now, we encourage you to buy one, so you'll be ready. Step counters are available at many sporting goods stores and online.

Here are a few features to look for when choosing a step counter:

- **Look for a device that only counts steps.** Devices that convert steps into miles and calories burned aren't accurate. Simple step counters, on the other hand, are reliable, as several studies have shown (Schenider et al. 2003, Schenider et al. 2004). They're also less expensive.

- **The step counter should have a cover.** You'll reset your step counter each morning, but in the meantime there is nothing more frustrating than bumping the reset button in the middle of the day. A cover will protect you from accidently losing your step count.

- **Look for a step counter with a leash.** Step counters are worn at your waist and can fall off. Choose one that has a string that tethers the device to a belt loop or waistband.

Weighing In

Maintaining a healthy weight depends on striking a healthy balance between what you eat and how active you are. Sometimes when people know how many calories a food contains—and how much activity it takes to burn off those calories—they have an easier time resisting temptations. Here's the amount of activity required for a 160-pound (72.6 kg) person to burn off excess calories equivalent to two popular foods. Go to the ALED Online Web site for more information on the amount of activity needed to burn the calories in common foods.

	Min of activity to burn off calories	
	Glazed donut (242 calories)	French fries, large order (400 calories)
Watching TV	186	308
Walking, 20 min per mi (1.6 km) pace	58	95
Scrubbing floors	54	89
Dancing (polka, line, country)	42	70
Bicycling, 12-14 mph (19.3-22.5 kph)	24	39
Running, 9 min per mi (1.6 km) pace	17	28

Real Life

Jerome participated in our Project *Active* study—sort of. Assigned to the lifestyle group, he attended the weekly meetings as requested. After about eight weeks, though, he stopped coming altogether. We continued to send him the educational materials. We also tried to reach him by phone on numerous occasions. He was a no-show for most of our assessment visits.

After the study was over and the scientific papers about the study were being published, we invited the Project *Active* participants back to The Cooper Institute for an appreciation party. Much to our surprise, Jerome showed up. What's more, he looked great! Turns out he was diagnosed with diabetes, and that scared him enough to start changing his lifestyle. He dug out all the Project *Active* materials and worked through them on his own. He told us, "I did everything you told me to do."

We learned something useful from Jerome. Even when it seems that people are not currently interested in changing, they will change when they are ready. Of course, it helps to be prepared with tools and information. So even if you're not ready to do all the activities in this book, continue to read through it. You never know when a story or idea might be the trigger to getting active for a lifetime.

? Did You Know?

It's never too late to make a change for the better. Studying a group of adults aged 65 and older, researchers at the Brigham and Women's Hospital and Harvard Medical School found that those who engaged in moderate- or vigorous-intensity physical activity had 28 to 44 percent lower mortality. They also enjoyed up to 53 percent more years of healthy life. Modern medicine has done an unprecedented job of increasing our life spans, and a healthier lifestyle, including good nutrition and physical activity, can help ensure that the extra time we have is quality time (Mozaffarian 2004).

Need a Boost?

Don't fret if you're having a hard time keeping up and meeting your goals. We all move forward at our own pace. Try these tips to help stay on track:

- Review the material in the previous weeks to find ideas that can help you meet your activity goals.
- Find a friend or family member who can encourage you to increase your activity.
- Remember that doing something is better than doing nothing. Try to fit in short bouts of activity whenever you can.
- Find ways to make physical activities fun. Do things you like to do with people you enjoy.
- Physical activity means moving instead of standing, sitting, or lying down. Take a few minutes to think about ways to replace inactive time with moving time.

The Confidence Factor

We've all heard that little voice in our heads that says, "I can't" or "I won't." On other occasions, we've heard a confident, self-assured voice say, "Of course I can. No problem." In the remainder of this chapter, we want you to consider ways to silence the negative voice and replace it with a positive one. We want you to turn "I can't" into "I know I can and will."

Here's another phrase we'd like you to use as often as possible: "I'll give it a try." To become active, especially if you've been sedentary for a while, it's important to try new activities, even if you're not sure you'll like them. To change anything about your life, you need to take some chances. You have to be willing to go out on a limb and take on new challenges. If you find yourself feeling reluctant, shake off your doubts and say to yourself, "I'll give it a try."

Countering Negative Arguments

Let's start by considering a few of the top reasons *not* to get up and do something active. Some we've talked about before, and at least one is probably a reason you've used yourself. For every one of the negatives, there's a good counterargument.

"I'm Too Tired to Move."

We've all used this excuse as a reason for flopping on the couch and not moving for the rest of the evening. Consider this: Physical activity usually makes people feel energized. Many volunteers in our program reported feeling invigorated after walking or taking a bicycle out for a spin. If you're too tired to move, the best remedy is usually to get up and move. You will nearly always feel better afterward.

"It's Been a Stressful Day, and I'm in a Rotten Mood."

We've all been there. Stress can wear most of us down. But the worst thing you can do is sit and fret. Dozens of studies have shown that physical activity is a great way to relieve stress and blow off the frustrations of the day. Most people report feeling happy and relaxed after a game of tennis, a soothing swim, or a walk around the neighborhood. Another plus: You'll experience the satisfaction of meeting your activity goal.

"I Have Way Too Much Work to Do."

Before you scuttle your plan to be active, consider this: taking a short activity break could improve your productivity. When people work without a break, productivity usually begins to slump. Get up from your desk for a five-minute walk. Climb a few flights of stairs. Take a walk around the block at lunch. Chances are you'll return feeling focused and full of energy to get the job done.

"It's Too Cold (or Hot or Rainy or Snowy) to Go Outside."

That's why it's important to have a backup plan. If you don't feel like walking outside, consider walking in the mall. If the weather is so bad you'd rather not drive to a mall, find a few things to do around the house. Options include simple calisthenics, jumping rope, or some heavy-duty housecleaning. If cold or rainy weather is a fact of life where you live, be ready with the clothes you need to brave the elements. Waterproof warm-up suits can keep you dry. Down jackets, gloves, and hats keep you warm. Once you start moving, you'll hardly notice the cold weather.

"I Want to Watch My Favorite TV Program Tonight."

Go ahead. Enjoy. Watching your favorite TV show, however, doesn't have to mean being inactive. Some volunteers in our programs used a rowing machine or a stationary bike while watching television. Others made a point of getting up during the commercials to stretch, take a quick walk, climb the stairs, or do a few calisthenics. Another strategy is to schedule a 10-minute walk before and after your favorite program. Right there you've tallied up 20 minutes. If your goal is to get 30 minutes of activity every day, another 10 minutes should be easy to find.

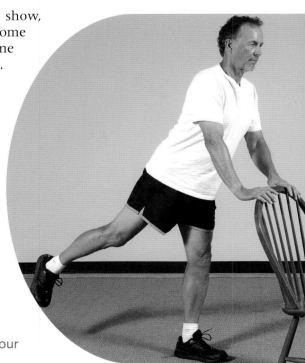

Our point is simple: For every good reason not to be active, there's an even better reason to get up and do something. To build confidence and encourage yourself, use positive messages to counteract the negative thoughts that sometimes get in your way.

You can get a good workout in the privacy of your home, even by exercising during commercials!

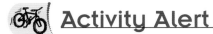

Activity Alert

Confidence Building

Here's a list of some of the challenges that keep people from being active. Overcoming challenges like these helps build confidence. You can also download a copy of this form from the ALED Online Web site.

Accentuating the Positive

Read the following negative messages. Circle the ones that you've said to yourself. Then write down at least one counterargument that accentuates the positive.

1. I don't want to do anything when I feel tired or down in the dumps.

_____

_____

_____

2. I don't know how to get started.

_____

_____

_____

3. I don't have anyone to be active with me.

_____

_____

_____

4. I can't find the time in my busy schedule.

_____

_____

_____

5. I'm going on vacation.

_____

_____

_____

6. I'm having a personal crisis.

_____

_____

_____

7. I just can't remember to exercise.

_____

_____

_____

8. I'm too sore from the last time.

_____

_____

_____

9. My family and friends don't support me.

_____

_____

_____

10. I haven't been feeling well all week.

_____

_____

_____

11. I'm discouraged because I never seem to reach my activity goal.

_____

_____

_____

12. I don't like to be active in public because I'm embarrassed by the way I look.

_____

_____

_____

13. I have back or knee problems that get in the way of being active.

_____

_____

_____

14. I get seasonal allergies and can't exercise outdoors.

_____

_____

_____

15. I don't feel safe exercising in my neighborhood.

_____

_____

_____

From S.N. Blair, A.L. Dunn, B.H. Marcus, R.A. Carpenter, and P. Jaret, 2011, _Active Living Every Day_, 2nd ed. (Champaign, IL: Human Kinetics).

If we've missed the negative message that gets in your way, write it down. How can you replace the negative with a positive?

Real Life

As a kid, Brenda could never live up to her parents' high expectations for her. Even as an adult, she still heard their voices in her head saying, "Why can't you try a little harder?" and "You'll never be a success if this is the best you can do." Those negative messages were especially loud when she looked at herself in the mirror and saw an overweight and out-of-shape reflection staring back at her.

When Brenda joined Project *Active*, she'd all but given up on becoming an active person. At first, all our work didn't shake that pessimistic idea. Then Brenda sat down with a sheet of paper and listed the problems that kept getting in her way. Often she couldn't find the support she needed. There were times when she felt too tired and sad to be active. Her busy schedule left her little time to be active.

For each of these challenges, she came up with an encouraging counterstatement. Sure, she sometimes had trouble finding support from her husband. But if she set her mind to it, she could do it on her own. Yes, her moods sometimes got in the way. But getting out and walking briskly often lifted her spirits and made her feel happy. True, her work schedule was sometimes crazy. With a little planning, however, she could always find 10 minutes here, 10 minutes there. Whenever a negative message threatened to overwhelm her resolve, Brenda reminded herself of the positive countermessage. Each time she did so, her confidence increased.

Celebrating Small Victories

Confidence comes from setting a goal, making a plan, and achieving it. Unfortunately, we often neglect to celebrate our own victories. That's especially true for people who have tried and failed before. All they can see is failure.

During the past few weeks, hopefully you've been able to meet your personal goals more than once. Over time, those small steps can add up to real success. Take a moment now and review what you've accomplished so far. Look back over the previous chapters and the goals you've set for yourself. Sure, you may not have scored 100 percent each week; few people do. Every small advance means progress.

Did You Know?

A century ago, most people couldn't help but get plenty of exercise. Household chores such as washing, cleaning, and ironing required hard physical labor. Working on a farm or in a factory meant working up a sweat. People walked to town and back instead of jumping into a car. In countless ways, the labor-saving devices of the 20th century have vastly improved the way we live and work. Factories have become wonders of automation. Thanks to farm machinery, farmers can create high yields that feed the earth's burgeoning population. Cars and planes have put once remote or inaccessible places within reach.

However, recently researchers have begun to see an unexpected drawback. The human body, it turns out, is built to be active. Our muscles need to lift and pull to remain strong. Our hearts need to beat fast once in a while to stay healthy. Our lungs need to exert themselves to promote stamina. Without physical activity, the risk of developing chronic diseases begins to climb. No one is suggesting we turn back the wheels of progress, but the latest findings on physical activity and health make it clear that we must find new ways to incorporate activity into everyday life.

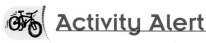 ## Activity Alert

Turning Errands Into Activity

Whether we're picking up groceries for dinner, stopping by the post office, or going to the bank, most of us run at least a few errands every day. Unfortunately, we don't really run. We don't even walk. We drive or take the bus. We wait in line. We get back in the car and drive home. Such day-to-day errands represent great opportunities for increasing your activity. All it takes is a little planning. For starters, make a list of the typical errands you run during the week. Some you may do every day; others, just once a week. Include everything that comes to mind.

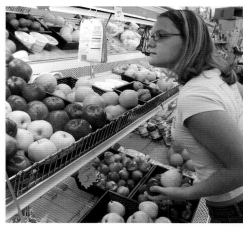

Which of your errands can you turn into physical activites?

A Week's Worth of Errands

1. _____
2. _____
3. _____
4. _____
5. _____

From S.N. Blair, A.L. Dunn, B.H. Marcus, R.A. Carpenter, and P. Jaret, 2011, *Active Living Every Day*, 2nd ed. (Champaign, IL: Human Kinetics).

Look over the list. Select two or three errands that, with a little tweaking, you could turn into physical activities. Let's say you typically drive to the grocery store, even though it's only five blocks from home. Walking there and back is a great opportunity to add 15 minutes of exercise and burn around 75 calories. Sure there are times when it's not practical to walk, especially when you have to pick up a lot of groceries. If you need just a few things for dinner, however, walking is a great alternative.

The same goes for errands to the bank or post office. Live too far to walk? Select a place several blocks from your destination to park the car or get off the bus and then walk the rest of the way. Choose a path that's pleasant and interesting to add another incentive. Over the next week, carry out your plan to turn a few errands into activities. If you keep a daily to-do list, add a star to the errands you've selected as physical activities to serve as a reminder.

CHAPTER CHECKLIST

Before you move on to the next week's activities, make sure you've done the following:

- Identified activities that are moderate and vigorous
- Estimated your walking pace
- Identified how you can burn 1,000 extra calories per week
- Ordered or purchased a step counter
- Identified negative messages that keep you from being physically active
- Turned at least two errands into opportunities for activity

 Checked out chapter 5 on the ALED Online Web site for more helpful resources and information for this chapter

References

Department of Health and Human Services. 2008. *Physical activity guidelines for Americans.* Washington, DC: Government Printing Office.

Hu, F.B., et al. 1999. Walking compared with vigorous physical activity and risk of type 2 diabetes in women: A prospective study. *Journal of the American Medical Association* 282(15): 1433-9.

Mozaffarian, D. 2004. Lifestyles of older adults: Can we influence cardiovascular risk in older adults? *American Journal of Geriatric Cardiology* 13(3): 153-160.

Schneider, P.L., et al. 2003. Accuracy and reliability of 10 pedometers for measuring steps over a 400-m walk. *Medicine and Science in Sports and Exercise* 35(10): 1179-1784.

Schneider, P.L., et al. 2004. Pedometer measures of free-living physical activity: Comparison of 13 models. *Medicine and Science in Sports and Exercise* 36(2): 331-334.

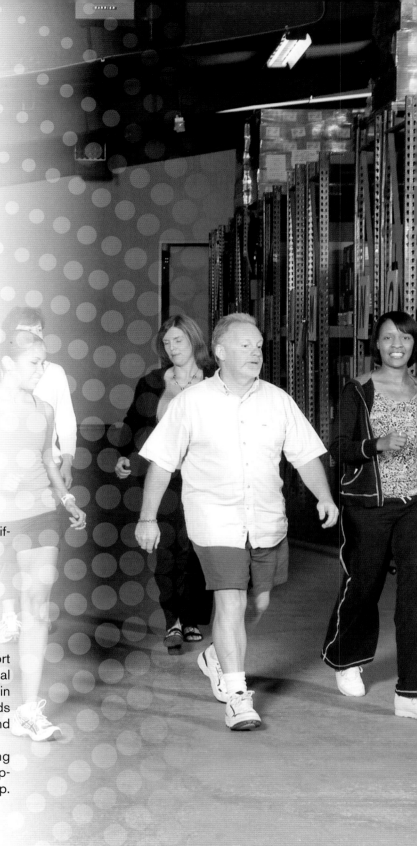

Chapter Six

Enlisting Support

In This Chapter

- Identifying key sources of support
- Spotting people who may make things difficult
- Learning how to ask for help
- Revisiting earlier activities
- Learning a few stretching techniques
- Assessing your progress so far

We are social animals. We thrive with the support of people around us. Research shows that social support is crucial to making a successful change in your life. The more supportive your family and friends are, the more likely you are to succeed in any kind of change.

Not all of us are surrounded by encouraging friends and family, of course. If you don't have support at home, there are other places to turn for help.

Finding the Support You Need

There are all kinds of support and all kinds of people who can offer it to you. Here are some examples:

- **A good listener.** This kind of help usually comes from people who listen to your triumphs and troubles without giving advice or making judgments about your thoughts or behavior. In other words, they're good sounding boards.

- **Someone who's been there.** This help comes from someone who's in the same boat as you are, knows what you're going through, and can sympathize with your feelings. People who've had similar experiences can usually offer helpful suggestions. Just knowing you're not the only one who has gone through something can be reassuring.

- **Someone who can offer knowledgeable advice.** Health professionals are a good source of information, and so are books, videos, newspapers, magazines, Web sites, or television. Be careful, though. Not all information is accurate or balanced. Some sources promote magic potions or products (the tip-off is when they ask you to send in $29.95 for some newfangled exercise device or diet breakthrough). Others offer quick fixes that are too good to be true.

- **An activity partner.** This help is offered by that special someone who's willing to join you on your morning walk or your bike ride after work. A walking or bicycling partner makes it easier to get out of bed on those mornings when you just don't feel like it. When someone else is depending on you for moral support, it's hard to blow it off and say no. Someone who offers to be a partner can give you that initial push you need to make activity a regular habit.

- **Someone who helps motivate you.** This kind of help comes from somebody who can pump up your determination or confidence—a cheerleader type who is upbeat, energetic, and enthusiastic.

- **Someone who offers emotional support.** This support is offered by someone who knows you and how you're feeling. Your happiness and well-being are all that matter to someone who offers genuine emotional support. A casual friend or coworker may offer good listening support, but real emotional support usually comes from a close friend or relative.

- **Someone who offers practical help.** This includes any help that makes it easier for you to succeed in making a lasting change in your life. It may be a spouse who takes on a few household chores to give you time for your walk after dinner or a grandparent who can sit with the kids while you go to a dance class.

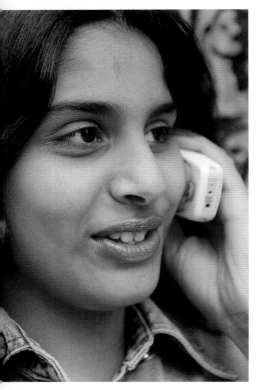

Friends can help to motivate you and offer emotional support.

Whom Can You Turn To?

You may not need all of these kinds of support all the time. At first, you may need shared experience to help you get past the early hurdles. Later you may get more out of practical support to help you stick to your goals. Remember, no single person is likely to offer all these forms of support (that person would have to be a saint). One person may be better at listening; another may be better at discussing shared experiences.

Support can come from many people around you, such as your kids. Look for opportunities to play with them, take a walk together, or engage in other active pursuits. Your spouse or significant other can also help. An early-morning or after-dinner walk is a great way to spend time together, talk over the events of the day, and get in some activity. But don't count on your spouse or significant other to be your sole source of support, either. You might strain your relationship.

Real Life

Over the last two years, Marilyn tried to increase her activity. Often she succeeded—for a week or two. Then work or family got in the way and her resolve fizzled. One day she noticed that her neighbor Carol walked every morning before breakfast. Marilyn asked if she could join her. Carol was happy for the company, and Marilyn was glad to have someone to motivate her. Now, even on days when she's rushed or not in the mood, she knows Carol is waiting, and she's not about to let her down.

Did You Know?

In a survey of 1,000 nonexercisers commissioned by the President's Council on Physical Fitness and Sports and the Sporting Goods Manufacturers Association (SGMA), 59 percent said they would like to exercise more (President's Council on Physical Fitness and Sports and the Sporting Goods Manufacturers Association 1993). What did two out of five say would be the biggest motivator? A spouse or significant other who supported and encouraged them. Even better, said the respondents, was a friend or relative to exercise with them.

Just Ask!

How can you find the support you need? Just ask! Many of us are uneasy asking for help, either because we fear rejection or we see it as a sign of weakness. However, everyone needs help from time to time, and most people are happy to offer it. When you ask for support, be open and candid. Explain why you're trying to become more active and why the support of people around you is so important. Be specific about what would help most. It's not enough to say to your kids, "Hey, how about cutting me a little slack?" You'll get more help by telling them exactly what they can do—cooking dinner, for example, or cleaning up the kitchen after dinner so you have time for a half-hour walk.

Real Life

From her experience with making other changes in her life, Sharita knew she worked better when other people were around to support and encourage her. She also knew that there were many other women in her local church who were looking for a way to increase their physical activity.

After the first few weeks in our program, Sharita took the initiative and organized a walking club with other women from her church. They began to meet in the evenings to walk around a local high school track. Whenever a woman missed a session, she had to put a dollar in the kitty. At the end of three months, the walkers who showed up most often got to share the money from the kitty. The real reward, of course, was enjoyed by all of them: a little extra motivation to help them reach their goal to increase their activity. This is a great example of emotional, motivational, and partnering support all rolled into one.

 ## Activity Alert

Recruiting Your Support Troops

Use the form on this page to recruit your supporters. First, take a moment to think about the things that still get in your way, such as lack of time, not feeling motivated, or not knowing how to get started. Be as specific as possible about the type of support that would help you overcome these barriers. Then think about the best people to turn to for the help you need. After you've put together your list of supporters, make a plan to talk to them. You can also download a copy of this form from the ALED Online Web site.

My Support Troops

What do I need help with?	Who could help me?	How could they help?	How could I reward them for helping me?
Example: Remembering to fit in physical activity during the day	My coworker Susan or my friend Charles	Call me once a day to check on how much activity I have gotten.	Every two weeks, go to the movies—my treat.

Beware the Exercise Saboteurs

Unfortunately, you may encounter people who try to discourage you or even sabotage your plans to make a lifestyle change. Why would anyone want to scuttle your plans? Change is threatening, especially to those we're closest to. A spouse or significant other may interpret your decision to become physically active as a criticism of her or as dissatisfaction with the relationship. Your coworkers may feel threatened by your resolution to increase your activity, especially if they feel guilty about their own inactivity.

Lack of support can take many forms. A spouse may complain about the time you spend exercising or throw roadblocks in your path in hopes of derailing you. Your boss may try to sabotage your lunchtime walks by scheduling meetings at noon. Even the best-intentioned friends can make it tough. Say they want you to go to lunch with them and you decline. They may start pressuring you in friendly ways that could be hard to resist.

What can you do if you meet opposition? Be open and positive. At the same time, be firm about your determination. Reassure your significant other that increasing your activity doesn't threaten your relationship, and try to involve him in your activities. The same goes for your boss or coworkers. Explain why your decision to become active is important to you and why you need help making it happen. Be friendly and accommodating. If you don't want to go to lunch with coworkers today, for instance, take a rain check for another day.

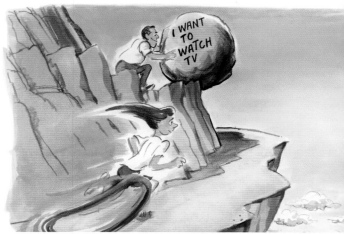

A Note on Naggers

It's good to offer support to people who are trying to make a change for the better. If you push them too hard, however, you may turn into a nag. Nagging is usually counterproductive. It can annoy and even discourage people from making healthy changes. Nagging often takes a negative or accusatory tone. Rather than make people feel empowered, it tends to make them feel as if they've failed.

If you're teaming up with someone to be more active, how can you make sure your efforts to encourage them don't turn into nagging? Here are a few tips:

- **Always adopt a positive tone.** Don't say, "Why didn't you show up for our walk yesterday?" Instead, say, "I really missed your company yesterday. Is everything OK?"
- **Look forward, not back.** Don't say, "You haven't shown up three times in the past two weeks." Instead, say, "What realistic goal can we set for next week?"
- **Offer constructive help.** Ask, "Is there anything I can do to help make things easier for you?"
- **Make it clear you care.** Say, "I really want you to reach your goal because I know it's important to you."

Real Life

Tony joined our program out of concern for not only his own health but also his family's well-being. He was particularly worried about his and his wife's inactivity and the message their inactivity conveyed to their kids. He had his heart set on taking walks with his wife. When she refused, he became discouraged. It was more than just a refusal. When he persisted, she began to ridicule his efforts. Fortunately, he recognized that he was only making things worse by insisting. So he turned elsewhere for support. He began talking to his coworkers at the warehouse about walking at lunchtime, and he found several who agreed to walk around the nearby mall with him. (It turned out that they had also been looking for ways to become active.) Of course, he still hopes his wife will eventually join him. For now, however, he doesn't depend solely on her support to work on his goal of being active.

 ## Activity Alert

Solo or With a Group

Would you prefer to be on your own when it comes to a more active lifestyle? That's great. Many people prefer exercising on their own. Still, consider turning to people around you for support and encouragement. Tell a friend or family member about your plan to become active, and explain how you hope to carry it out. Chances are good this person will ask you now and then, "How's your bike riding (walking, swimming) going?". The fact that someone cares will help keep you motivated. If you're a go-it-alone person, use the following blanks to write down the names of two or three people who could encourage you:

1. _____
2. _____
3. _____

From S.N. Blair, A.L. Dunn, B.H. Marcus, R.A. Carpenter, and P. Jaret, 2011, *Active Living Every Day*, 2nd ed. (Champaign, IL: Human Kinetics).

If you thrive on companionship, take a few minutes this week to check out activity clubs in your area. Most places have groups that get together to walk, run, cycle, skate, hike, swim, or dance (ballroom, country and western, tap, swing, and so on). Check out your local recreation department online or look in the newspaper. Use the following blank lines to put together a list of what you discover. If you don't find what you're looking for, consider starting your own group of lunchtime walkers or after-work bikers by posting a message at the office cafeteria, your church, the local recreation center, or online social networking sites.

1. _____
2. _____
3. _____

From S.N. Blair, A.L. Dunn, B.H. Marcus, R.A. Carpenter, and P. Jaret, 2011, *Active Living Every Day*, 2nd ed. (Champaign, IL: Human Kinetics).

Social Support at a Distance

Modern technology offers a novel way to find social support at a distance, as one of the authors of this book discovered firsthand. Steve Blair, who has been a runner for over 40 years, still manages to run nearly every day. A year ago, after joining a research project based at the University of Pennsylvania, he joined a pedometer group whose members send each other an e-mail each day tallying up how many steps they've taken. The messages are simple—for example, "Steve 12,576 Monday." After joining the group, Steve decided to set a goal of taking 5 million steps in his 70th year.

As of this writing, he is more than one-quarter of the way through the year and is well ahead of schedule. A good part of the reason for his success is the social support he receives via the daily e-mails. Steve already knew support was important for participants in the ALED program. Still, he was surprised at how powerful it has proved to be for someone like him, who is already quite active. Perhaps even more surprising, Steve only knows a half a dozen members of the steps group. He has never met most of them—the group is scattered around the world. The point is that you can use modern technology such as e-mail, text messaging, Facebook, Twitter, or other means of communication to take reap the benefits of social support.

Did You Know?

Take a stroll in the morning or the early evening in the Brazilian city of Recife, the fifth largest city in Brazil, and you're likely to see lots of people exercising. In 2002, city officials launched a program that offers free exercise classes in 21 public spaces. Physical education instructors teach calisthenics and dance classes to all comers, and the residents of Recife have been flocking to join in. Since the program began, more than 100,000 people have enrolled each year and have participated in 888,000 exercise classes. A new study of the program also shows that current and past participants are three times more likely than those who never participated to continue leading physically active lives. The free classes, in other words, seem to inspire people to make lasting changes for the better.

Real Life

When Barry joined our program, inactivity wasn't his only worry. He'd gone through a difficult divorce, and he was having trouble with his teenage son, who felt angry and confused. A week after he began a walking plan, Barry decided to invite his son to join him for a brisk walk before dinner. The boy was reluctant, but he finally agreed. Because he didn't know how to fix dinner for himself, he figured he had no choice. Their walks were quiet at first. After a while, though, they began talking. Gradually their conversations became more intimate. They began to talk about their feelings about the divorce and what lay ahead. Adding a simple activity to family life gave Barry a benefit he never expected.

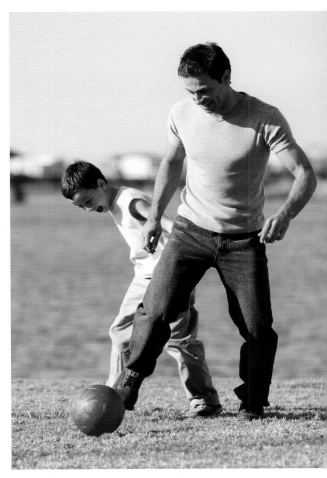

Exercising with family members can bring unexpected benefits.

Taking Stock of What You've Accomplished

Nobody learns everything the first time around. The process of becoming an expert at anything usually requires going through certain steps again and again. Along the way we gain understanding.

Think back to your "Aha!" moments, those times when you've suddenly had a big insight. Often they arrive after you've mulled over the same problem many times. Recall what it's like to return to one of your favorite books or movies and discover things you never noticed were there.

The same concept applies when you're trying to change. Often you need to try things several times before you fully understand their value. That's why we think it's worthwhile to revisit some earlier territory. We've selected three activities from previous chapters that are well worth repeating.

 ## Activity Alert

Three Easy Activities

In addition to what you're doing to meet the goals you've set for yourself, we'd like you to do three simple activities. You can do them in any order. If you're worried about finding the time, sit down with your calendar and schedule each activity in advance.

1. Walk, don't drive.

This one's easy: Go shopping. Instead of circling the block or cruising the parking lot to find the nearest parking place, park your car at a distance and walk briskly to the store. If you don't drive, get off the bus or subway at least one stop before the shopping area and walk. While you're walking, look around and try to find something you hadn't noticed before—a new shop window, a particularly beautiful tree, even an interesting crack in the sidewalk. Add up the extra time you spend walking.

2. Find some company.

At least once this week, turn a few minutes with a friend, family member, or coworker into an opportunity for activity. Suggest a walk in a nearby park or shopping mall. Plan a walk-and-talk business meeting. If the weather is good, how about a spin on a bike? (Don't forget to wear a helmet!)

3. Watch TV.

This may be the easiest of all: Watch TV. That's right—set aside an evening to watch a few of your favorite programs. Here's the catch: Instead of vegging out during those long commercial breaks, walk around the house (or the block), dance to some music, or do some serious cleaning—anything that qualifies as moderate-intensity activity. Add up the extra minutes you spend being active.

Troubleshooting: Getting Nowhere Fast?

If you're finding it hard to push yourself toward achieving your goal, it's time for a little problem solving. First, be honest with yourself. Have you been doing 150 minutes of moderate-intensity activity weekly for several weeks? If not, you may need to work on being more consistent. Consistency is the key to building fitness.

If you have met the weekly goal of 150 minutes for several weeks, then it's time to check your pace. You may need to pick up the intensity a little to increase your fitness level. Don't go gangbusters; simply try to increase your pace a little each week. Use a watch to record your time, if that helps, or monitor how winded you feel at the end of your activity. Push yourself a little harder each time, and it won't be long before you see a difference.

Stretching Exercises

So far, we've focused on activities that burn calories and improve fitness. What about activities that increase flexibility, such as stretching exercises or yoga? Some athletes believe that doing stretching exercises before a workout reduces the risk of injury. So far, there's not much scientific evidence to support that idea. And stretching is not going strengthen your heart and muscles. But that doesn't mean it's not important. We're convinced that stretching exercises help people stay active by keeping joints and muscles flexible. Obviously, maintaining the ability to reach and bend is important in everyday life.

With that in mind, we offer four easy stretching exercises you can do when you first wake up or between TV commercials.

Achilles Tendon and Calf Stretch

This exercise stretches the heel cord and the back of the lower leg. Stand 2 or 3 feet (61-91 cm) from a wall or tree with both toes pointed forward as you lean toward the wall with your left leg forward with knee slightly bent and your right leg in back and straight, partly supporting yourself with your hands. Keep both heels flat to stretch the calf. Hold 10 to 20 seconds, and repeat.

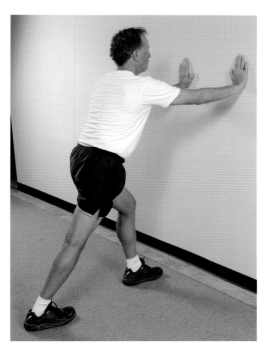

Achilles tendon and calf stretch.

Hurdler Stretch

This exercise stretches the muscles of the back of the thigh. From a seated position bend your left knee and place the sole of left foot on the inside of your right knee (see photo). With your right knee very slightly bent, lean over your right leg, reaching toward your toes on your right foot. Keep your head and back straight as you move into the stretch. Hold 10 to 20 seconds, and repeat. Switch legs and repeat again.

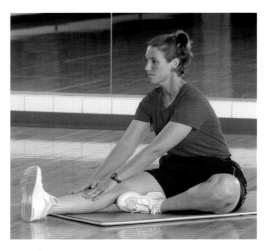

Hurdler stretch.

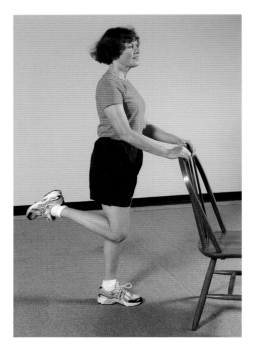

Modified quadriceps stretch.

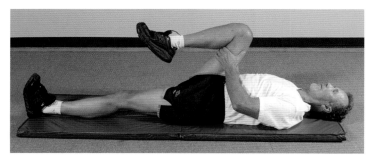

Lower-back stretch.

Quadriceps Stretch

This exercise stretches the muscles of the front of the thigh. Place your left hand against a chair, wall, or tree for balance and then grab your right ankle with your right hand and pull it up and back toward your buttocks until you can feel a stretch in the front of your right thigh. Or you can simply bend your leg back and toward your buttocks (see photo). Keep your back straight and your right knee pointing toward the ground. The standing leg should have a slightly bent knee. Hold the stretch for 10 to 20 seconds, and repeat with the left leg.

Lower-Back Stretch

This exercise stretches the muscles of the lower back. Lie flat on the floor on your back with your legs extended, and pull the right knee up to your chest. Bend your left knee slightly and press your back to the ground. Hold the position 10 to 20 seconds, and repeat with the left knee.

Keep in mind that time spent on stretching exercises doesn't count toward meeting your activity goals. Still, these exercises are a great way to get ready for activity or to cool down afterward. They're also a great way to relax if you find yourself under stress.

The Yoga Option

Yoga is one of the oldest physical disciplines in the world. The age-old practice combines meditation, breathing exercises, and postures that are thought to focus physical and mental energy. Yoga has been shown to have many health benefits. These include reducing stress and anxiety and easing depression. Yoga is typically not an aerobic activity, so it doesn't count toward meeting exercise recommendations for moderate activity. But some forms of yoga do improve muscle strength and flexibility and thus can help you stay active and healthy.

Yoga has been around for so long that a variety of forms have evolved:

- **Hatha yoga**—the traditional practice of postures designed to improve flexibility, balance, and strength while focusing the mind and body
- **Ashtanga yoga**—sometimes called *power yoga* because it emphasizes powerful movements that require strength and stamina
- **Iyengar yoga**—a combination of slow, controlled movements
- **Kundalini yoga**—rapid movements accompanied by meditation, chanting, and breathing exercises
- **Bikram yoga**—popularly known as *hot yoga* because it is performed in warm rooms in order to boost flexibility

Most practitioners combine several approaches. For information on yoga classes, check out your local fitness centers or community recreation programs. You'll also find useful information from the American Yoga Association at www.americanyogaassociation.org and from Yoga in Canada at www.yogadirectorycanada.com.

Did You Know?

What's the best remedy for an aching back? According to a 2009 study funded by the National Institutes of Health, most chronic back pain sufferers don't know the answer, in large part because their doctors aren't telling them. Many trials have shown that exercise effectively eases chronic back pain, improves function, and minimizes disability. Yet when researchers at the University of North Carolina at Chapel Hill surveyed almost 700 people with chronic back pain, less than half had been prescribed exercise. Of those who were, 46 percent were given an exercise prescription by a physical therapist, 27 percent by a physician, and 21 percent by a chiropractor. Based on the evidence, the scientists concluded that more people with chronic back and neck pain should be encouraged to exercise as a way to relieve their discomfort.

Activity Alert

How Are You Doing?

Now that the first six sessions are almost done, it's time for a progress report. You've likely had some new insights about how you spend your time, and you've come up with some great ideas to turn sedentary time into active time. Take a few minutes to think about the following questions. We encourage you to write out your answers. Keeping a record of your progress and your thoughts along the way can help you look back and see how far you've come.

1. Which activities do you enjoy the most?

2. Which activities do you enjoy the least? Why?

3. Have you achieved at least one of your goals? If not, what has gotten in your way?

4. Has your attitude toward physical activity changed? If so, how?

5. Have you tried any new activities? If not, list one that you might want to try in the second half of the program.

6. Are you still challenged by negative thoughts about yourself and activity? If so, what are they? What positive messages can you use to counter them?

From S.N. Blair, A.L. Dunn, B.H. Marcus, R.A. Carpenter, and P. Jaret, 2011, *Active Living Every Day*, 2nd ed. (Champaign, IL: Human Kinetics).

Need a Boost?

Having a hard time meeting your goals? Never fear. Everyone encounters obstacles now and then. Here are some tips that can help you keep on track:

- Look back over the material in the previous week or two to find ideas or strategies to help you meet your activity goals.
- Post a list of physical activity benefits in a conspicuous place, such as the refrigerator, the TV, or your car dashboard.
- Visualize yourself as an active person. Think about how you'll spend your time and how you'll feel. Imagine the benefits you'll gain from increasing your activity.
- Ask someone close to you to help you come up with solutions to the issues that are holding you back.
- Remember, becoming active for life is a process—it's not something you can expect to do overnight. Be patient. Set small goals.
- Give yourself a break. If you can't keep up, take the pace a little slower. Spend two weeks on a chapter.
- Keep track of your plans, goals, and activities. Keeping an activity log or wearing a pedometer is a powerful motivator.
- Resolve to put activity high on your list of priorities. If you're not convinced, look back over the benefits of an active life that mean the most to you.

CHAPTER CHECKLIST

Before you move on to the next week's activities, make sure you've done the following:

- Specified the kind of help you need most
- Identified two or three people who can support you in your effort to become active
- Identified ways to help your support troops in return
- Practiced a few stretching exercises
- Reviewed your progress so far
- **Checked out chapter 6 on the ALED Online Web site for more helpful resources and information for this chapter**

References

President's Council on Physical Fitness and Sports and the Sporting Goods Manufacturers Association. 1993. American attitudes toward physical activity and fitness: A national survey. A survey conducted by Peter D. Hart Research Associates. Washington, D.C.

Chapter Seven

Avoiding Pitfalls

In This Chapter

- Recognizing the all-or-nothing trap
- Identifying pitfalls that can trip you up
- Planning for high-risk situations
- Adding a few muscle-strengthening activities

The best intentions aren't always enough. Sometimes your determination will falter. Maybe you do fine until the holidays hit and your schedule goes awry. Maybe you're on track to reach your goal until a hectic stretch at work or a rocky phase in a relationship gets in the way. Maybe you injure yourself or come down with the flu.

Whatever the reason, there are times when it's tough to stick to your plan for physical activity. In this chapter we'll look at strategies to deal with the rough times. The goal is to avoid letting a brief lapse turn into a longer relapse or a full-fledged collapse.

The All-or-Nothing Trap

One of the first mistakes people make when they fall short of their goal is to think, "That's it. I've blown it. I'll never make this work. Maybe I'm just destined to be a couch potato."

Don't believe it. A one-time slip doesn't mean you're a failure. It doesn't mean you're fated to be inactive forever. That's the all-or-nothing trap. Plenty of people with the best intentions have fallen into it. They mistakenly think, "Either I stick to my plan and meet my goal, or I'm a failure."

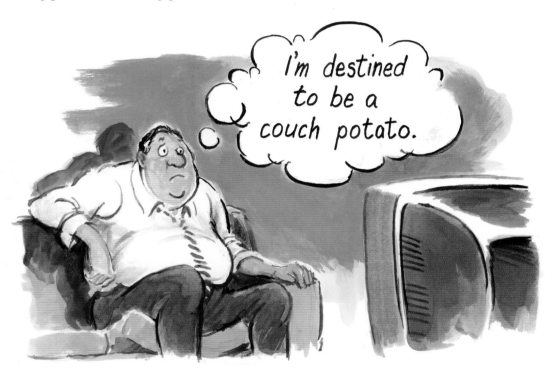

All-or-nothing thinking is taking the easy way out. It's a fancy way of quitting. Okay, so you've missed a day or two of activity. Maybe you've blown a whole week. Maybe you've been out of commission for a month or more. The important point is to understand it for what it is: a lapse. Sure, you've fallen behind. But all is not lost. Remind yourself of all you've learned. Think about how far you've come since you started. Look back through this book if you need proof that you've made progress. With a little effort, you can take two steps forward and keep up the progress you've been making.

One thing you don't want to do is give up. The key to recovering from a lapse is to act fast. Here's what to do:

- **Be honest.** Admit to yourself that you've hit a snag. Figure out exactly how long you've lapsed and think about what knocked you off track. Look at lapses not as failures but as learning opportunities.

- **Turn to your support troops.** If you've gotten support and encouragement from friends or loved ones, turn to them for another pep talk. No one likes to admit that they've faltered. By telling someone, however, you may be able to enlist help to get out of the rut and back on track. Turn back to chapter 6 for ideas on getting support.

- **Start planning immediately.** Return to the Personal Time Study form on page 8. If your schedule has changed significantly since your last time study, complete the form again for a couple of days. The goal is to identify opportunities to fit in activity. Put them in your calendar.

- **Set new goals.** Think about ways you might revise your plans and goals to make them work better for you. Try to incorporate activities that you enjoy. Set a date when you will start again. You may need to work up slowly to the level you were at before. That's fine. The important thing is to commit to a goal of getting back into an active lifestyle. Give yourself a little time, and you'll regain all the lost ground.

- **Avoid negative messages.** Remember those discouraging voices that sometimes speak up when things go wrong—the voices that say things such as "failure," "can't," or "never"? Counter those negative messages with positive ones. Instead of saying, "I can't stick to my plan," remind yourself that you did fine for the first month. Make a new plan for what you can do from now on.

- **Focus on your strengths.** Look back over a time when you were doing well. Think about the personal strengths you discovered. Perhaps you learned that you like doing activities with other people. Maybe you found that you achieve more if you have a specific plan and a schedule for meeting your goal. Similar to some participants in our program, you may have discovered that you enjoy certain activities, such as dancing, cycling, or walking your dog. Enjoying activities is an important strength you can leverage. Once you've identified your personal strengths, think about ways to use them now to get yourself back in the game.

Real Life

Fran and her husband Eddie were into their eighth week of walking 30 minutes after dinner every weeknight. They'd rediscovered the pleasures of seeing the neighborhood. They relished spending quiet time together. Fran had even begun to see an improvement in the mirror, and Eddie's doctor was pleased to see that his blood sugar levels were going down a little.

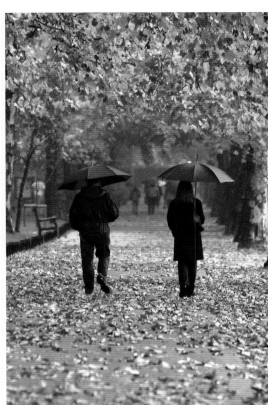

Then trouble struck. Lifting a heavy box, Fran wrenched her back. By the next morning she could barely get out of bed. She spent a week recuperating at home, and a month passed before the pain subsided enough to allow her to walk any distance at all. Eddie had to take on most of the household duties. He could see the frustration in Fran's face when she couldn't go walking. He didn't want to hurt her feelings by leaving her alone in the house while he walked.

For both of them, a lapse was beginning to turn into a full-fledged collapse. Fran was ready to give up completely when Eddie came to the rescue. He reminded her how much pleasure they'd gotten out of their walks. He convinced her that she would recover faster if she were active. They revised their goals to begin with a 10-minute walk and set a date on the calendar to begin again. For an added incentive, Eddie picked up a brand new pair of walking shoes for Fran. Within a month they were back to walking 30 minutes every evening.

Did You Know?

Many women gain weight during menopause. Those extra pounds, especially around the middle, increase the risk of heart disease. A University of Pittsburgh study published in the *Annals of Behavioral Medicine* showed that middle-aged women who took part in the 5-year Women's Healthy Lifestyle Project, which included both a healthier diet and more physical activity, kept their weight from climbing. Fifty-five percent remained at or below their starting weight, compared with only 26 percent of those in a control group. They kept their waistlines from expanding, too (Simkin-Silverman et al. 2003).

Trouble Ahead

Sometimes trouble comes out of nowhere—an injury, for example, or a family crisis. But more often, the potholes in the road are easy to predict. If you know what situations cause problems, you can avoid being ambushed by them. Here are three common high-risk situations and simple tips on how to steer clear of a lapse.

Emotional Upsets

Minor or major crises, even everyday stresses, can undermine your motivation. It's natural to think, "I'm too stressed to fit physical activity into my schedule right now." The solution: Remind yourself that being an inactive couch potato isn't going to improve the situation. In fact, going for a brief walk can help you feel better. Plus, it can give you time to come up with ways to counter stress.

Travel

When we find ourselves in a new setting and an unfamiliar schedule, it's easy to get distracted. The solution is to plan ahead. If you have a favorite pair of walking shoes, be sure to pack them. If there are no places to go for a walk at your hotel or you don't feel safe, check out other options: local shopping malls, city parks with walking paths, even the airport. Usually hotel staff can advise you about safe places to walk when you arrive. If the weather outside is frightful, use hotel hallways and stairs to walk and climb. Many hotels have pools, so be sure to pack a swimsuit. Even if you're not a regular swimmer, taking a plunge can be a great way to unwind after a long trip or an intense business meeting.

Vacations offer many opportunities to try something new, from playing Frisbee golf to snorkeling. Before you leave, make a list of physical activities you'll do while you're away. You may even want to plan a vacation around an activity, such as hiking in a state park or renting a bike and cycling at the beach. If you're visiting a large city, one of the best ways to see the sights is to follow a walking-tour map of interesting sites.

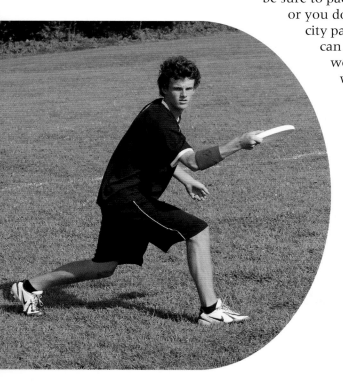

Even on vacations, you can find ways to be physically active.

Injuries and Health Problems

Some injuries and other medical problems are serious enough that you have to put physical activity on hold until you've recovered. But for garden-variety back problems or mild arthritis, being active can be just what the doctor ordered. (Always check with your doctor first, of course, if you have any questions.) After an injury, you may need to modify your activities so that you still get exercise. One avid bicyclist we know injured his shoulder and couldn't ride for a couple of months, but he discovered that he could use a stationary bike at the gym because he didn't need to steer it. When someone else we know sprained an ankle and had to stop walking temporarily, she took up swimming instead.

Weighing In

Holiday Weight Gain

Lots of food and little time to be active add up to extra pounds during the holidays, or so many of us have come to believe. But the dangers of holiday feasting may not be quite what you think. In a study published several years ago, people averaged only a 1-pound (.45 kg) weight gain during the holidays instead of 5 pounds (2.26 kg) as was previously thought. The bad news: They didn't lose what they'd gained. Thus, many years of small holiday weight gains add up! Planning to stay active during the holidays—and resolving to be more active after they're over—can prevent weight gain and combat holiday stress (Yanovski et al. 2000).

Did You Know?

Jumping on your bike for a spin around the neighborhood may lower your risk of one of the leading forms of cancer. In Norway, researchers found that as few as four hours of moderate cycling per week reduced the risk of colon cancer in female participants by almost 40 percent (Thune 1996).

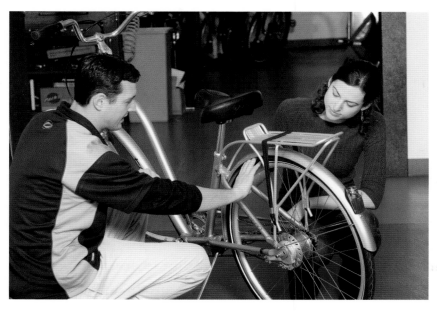

Your local bike shop can offer tips on equipment, local bike paths, and biking clubs.

Activity Alert

Planning for High-Risk Situations

There are plenty of obstacles out there. We have showed you how to solve some common challenges. Now it is your turn.

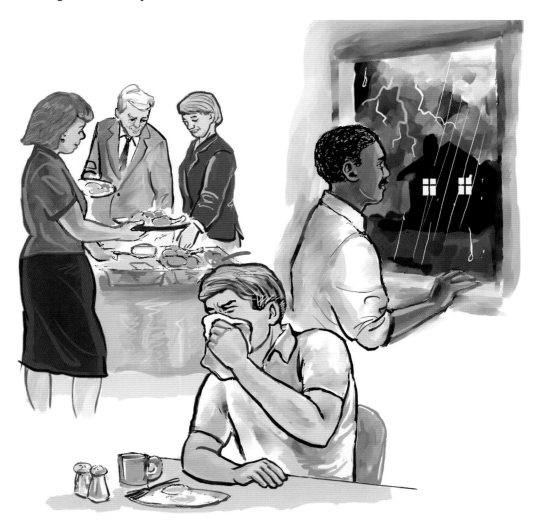

Following are high-risk situations that cause many people to falter. Check off those that are most likely to trip you up. Then go back and think about each situation. What does it feel like when you run into trouble? How could you plan to avoid trouble the next time it comes along? These tips will help:

1. **Define the problem by breaking it down into several manageable parts.**

2. **Formulate a plan that is specific and achievable.**

3. **Consider your strengths and resources, including friends, family, or resources in the community.**

You can also download a copy of this form from the ALED Online Web site.

Problem Solving for High-Risk Situations

Holiday madness

It's December. The entire family is coming to town for the holidays. You usually end up sitting around, eating too much, and getting almost no physical activity. The holidays have been your downfall before. What's the biggest problem you encounter?

_____

_____

What plan can you make now to stay on track and get more physical activity than you have in the past?

_____

_____

No time for yourself

It's been a busy week at work. There's no relief in sight. By the time you get home, you're exhausted. Your plans for physical activity are beginning to totter. What are your thoughts and feelings?

_____

_____

Physical activity is a terrific antidote to stress. What plan can you make to fit it in, even during the busiest times?

_____

_____

Poor weather

It's too cold (hot, snowy, rainy, humid) to go out and do anything. What are your thoughts at a time like this?

_____

_____

You can't buy the right weather, but you can buy the right gear or you can come up with alternatives that don't leave you out in the cold. What's your plan for dealing with foul weather?

_____

_____

Good Samaritan

You are unexpectedly called out of town to take care of a sick relative who has been hospitalized. You don't know how long you'll be gone. What are your thoughts and feelings about sticking with your plan for physical activity?

_____

_____

Physical activity can help you stay in a positive frame of mind and cope with life's challenges. What positive messages and physical activities can you come up with to keep yourself going?

_____

_____

From S.N. Blair, A.L. Dunn, B.H. Marcus, R.A. Carpenter, and P. Jaret, 2011, _Active Living Every Day_, 2nd ed. (Champaign, IL: Human Kinetics).

Did You Know?

People in lower-income neighborhoods are especially prone to sedentary lifestyles. Fears about safety may be one reason. In 2007, a team led by researchers at the Harvard School of Public Health interviewed 1,180 residents in low-income complexes in the Boston area. They used step counters to tally how many steps the respondents took. Most of the residents felt safe during the day, but almost two-thirds said they didn't feel safe at night. The men in the sample were just as active whether they felt safe or not. Women who felt unsafe at night, however, took many fewer steps—4,302 versus 5,178 (Bennett et al. 2007).

Many communities are doing things to make neighborhoods safer. They are also providing activity options that people can use without worry. But most cities and towns have not made changes to encourage healthier habits. In the meantime, if you feel unsafe at night, schedule your activity time during the day. If you can't do that, consider organizing a group of people to walk together in the evening. Contact your local recreation department. Another alternative is to find an indoor shopping mall where you can walk and feel safe.

Activity Alert

Preparing for High-Risk Situations

We've looked at how you can steer clear of high-risk situations by planning. Take a moment now to think about the activities, events, and situations that you will face in the next six months. List three that may put your physical activity efforts at risk. After each high-risk situation, list two or three things you can do to make sure it doesn't cause a lapse or a total collapse. You can also download a copy of this form from the ALED Online Web site.

Planning for High-Risk Situations

High-risk situation 1

_____

_____

How to avoid trouble

_____

_____

High-risk situation 2

_____

_____

_____

How to avoid trouble

_____

_____

_____

High-risk situation 3

_____

_____

_____

How to avoid trouble

_____

_____

_____

From S.N. Blair, A.L. Dunn, B.H. Marcus, R.A. Carpenter, and P. Jaret, 2011, *Active Living Every Day*, 2nd ed. (Champaign, IL: Human Kinetics).

Flexing Your Muscles

Activities such as walking and bicycling make your heart and lungs work more efficiently. But what about the muscles in your legs, arms, and back? Research shows that strengthening all the muscle groups through resistance training is also important to health. One reason is obvious: We use our muscles for all kinds of everyday activities, from getting out of chairs to lifting bags of groceries. Another reason may surprise you: Maintaining strong muscles helps bones stay strong. And it may help you better control your weight because muscle tissue burns calories even when you are sleeping. The more calories you burn, of course, the easier it is to keep weight off.

Maintaining muscular fitness can also help prevent falls, which are a leading cause of disability as we age (Paterson et al. 2007). In addition, recent studies show that people with low muscular strength are more likely to die prematurely than people who are stronger—and that older people who start exercising can lower their risk of dying prematurely (Portgjis et al. 2007). The health benefits of muscular strength are in addition to the health benefits of aerobic exercises, such as walking and biking. That's why the 2008 Physical Activity Guidelines for Americans recommend two days of resistance training each week (Department of Health and Human Services 2008).

We encourage you to begin trying out some muscle-strengthening exercises. Don't panic. Get started with these simple ways to give the major muscles groups in your body a workout. Don't worry if you don't have any dumbbells on hand for the upper-body exercises. Simply use a soup can, book, or other weighty object.

Upper-Body Exercises

Three simple exercises for upper-body resistance training are the seated biceps curl, the triceps kickback, and the chest press from the supine position.

Seated Biceps Curl

Adapted, by permission, from National Strength and Conditioning Association, 2008, *Exercise technique manual for resistance training*, 2nd Ed. (Champaign, IL: Human Kinetics), 138-39.

Following are the steps for the seated biceps curl.

Starting Position

- Grasp two equal-weight dumbbells with a closed, neutral grip.
- Lift the dumbbells off the floor, and sit on a chair or bench.
- Keep the upper body erect, shoulders held back, and eyes focused ahead.
- Allow the dumbbells to hang.

Upward Movement

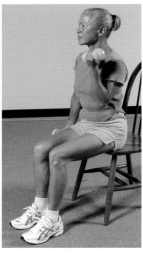

Seated biceps curl.

- Begin the exercise by raising one dumbbell upward by flexing the arm at the elbow. The nonexercising arm should be kept stationary at the side (only one arm is involved at a time).
- Keep the wrist stiff and the upper arm stationary against the side of the upper body as the dumbbell is raised; do not let it move forward or outward. No movement should occur at the shoulder; movement should occur only at the elbow joint.
- Flex the elbow with a neutral hand position as the little-finger half of the dumbbell passes by the thigh and moves to the front of the body. When this occurs, begin to rotate the forearm and wrist by turning the hand outward.
- Continue flexing the elbow and rotating the forearm and wrist until the dumbbell is near the shoulder in a palms-up hand position (see photo). If the elbow moves forward at the highest dumbbell position, then the elbow has flexed too far.

Downward Movement

- Lower the dumbbell slowly and under control to the starting position by gradually rotating the forearm and wrist by turning the hand inward.
- Keep the wrist stiff, the upper arm stationary against the side of the upper body, and the feet flat on the floor.
- Continue to lower the dumbbell until the elbow is fully extended but not locked.
- Repeat the upward and downward movement phases with the other arm. Continue to alternate the arms to complete the set.
- At the completion of the set, return the dumbbells to the floor in a controlled manner.

Triceps Kickback

Following are the steps for the triceps kickback.

Starting Position

- Stand on the right side of a flat bench with a dumbbell on the floor next to the right foot.

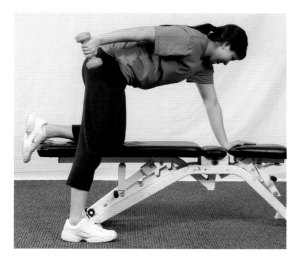

Triceps kickback.

- Kneel on the bench with the left leg, and lean forward to place the left hand on the bench in front of the left knee. Place the hand far enough ahead of the knee on the bench so that the left arm and left thigh are parallel to each other.
- The inside of the right thigh or knee should be very close to the right side of the bench, with the toes pointing ahead.
- Reach down with the right hand and grasp the dumbbell with a closed, neutral grip.
- Move the right arm to position the upper arm next to the upper body and parallel to the floor.
- Allow the dumbbell to hang.
- Slightly flex the right knee and maintain this flexed position during the exercise.

Upward Movement

- Extend the right elbow to lift the dumbbell until the whole arm is parallel to the floor (see photo).
- The upper right arm and elbow should be kept near the side of the body.
- Do not swing or jerk the upper body upward to help raise the dumbbell.

Downward Movement

- Lower the dumbbell slowly and under control to the starting position; do not allow the dumbbell to jerk the arm down.
- After completing a set with the right arm, set the dumbbell on the floor, stand on the left side of the bench, and repeat the exercise using the left arm.

Chest Press From Supine Position

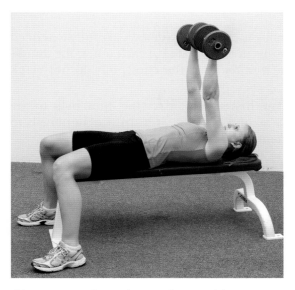

Chest press from the supine position.

Adapted, by permission, from National Strength and Conditioning Association, 2008, *Exercise technique manual for resistance training*, 2nd Ed. (Champaign, IL: Human Kinetics), 72-74.

Following are the steps for the chest press from the supine position.

Starting Position

- Grasp two equal-weight dumbbells with a closed grip. Position the outside surface of the little-finger half of the dumbbells against the front of the thighs (the dumbbell handles will be parallel to each other).
- Sit on one end of a flat bench with the dumbbells resting on the thighs.
- Lie back so the head rests on the other end of the bench. Move the dumbbells to the chest (armpit) area and then to an extended-elbow position above the chest with the forearms parallel to each other. Reposition the head, shoulders, buttocks, and feet to

achieve a five-point body-contact position: 1. Head is placed firmly on the bench. 2. Shoulders and upper back are placed firmly and evenly on the bench. 3. Buttocks are placed evenly on the bench. 4. Right foot is flat on the floor. 5. Left foot is flat on the floor.

- The most common dumbbell position is with the dumbbell handles in line with each other with the palms facing toward the feet. Another option is to hold the dumbbells in a neutral position (parallel to each other with the palms facing each other).

Downward Movement

- Begin the exercise by lowering the dumbbells slowly and under control toward the chest. To maintain a stable body position on the bench, lower the dumbbells at the same rate.
- Keep the wrists stiff, the forearms at a right angle to the floor, and the dumbbell handles in line with each other. Minimize all forward-to-backward and side-to-side movement.
- Guide the dumbbells down and slightly out to the sides of the chest, near the armpits. Visualize a bar passing through both dumbbell handles: the lowest position of the dumbbells is where the imaginary bar would touch the chest at nipple level.
- Do not arch the low back to raise the chest.
- Keep the head, upper body, hips, and feet in a five-point body-contact position.

Upward Movement

- Press the dumbbells upward at the same rate and very slightly toward each other to keep them under control.
- Maintain the same stationary five-point body-contact position; do not arch the low back or lift the buttocks or feet.
- Keep the wrists stiff, the forearms at a right angle to the floor, and the dumbbell handles in line with each other; do not allow the dumbbells to sway as they are raised.
- Continue pressing the dumbbells up until the elbows are fully extended (see photo). Keep the forearms nearly parallel to each other; the dumbbells can move toward each other over the chest, but do not clank them together.
- At the completion of the set, first slowly lower the dumbbells to the chest (armpit) area and then, one at a time, return the dumbbells to the floor in a controlled manner.

Back and Core Exercise

Two simple exercises for back and core resistance training are the back extension and the simple crunch or pelvic tilt.

Back Extension

Following are the steps for the back extension.

Starting Position

- Lie facedown on a floor mat.
- Place the toes on the floor 6 to 12 inches (15-30 cm) apart with the knees fully extended.
- Place the palms of the hands on the mat, rest the face on the back of the hands, and point the elbows out to the sides.

Upward Movement

- Begin the exercise by lifting the upper body slowly and under control.
- Keep the face in contact with the back of the hands; do not lift the upper body or head with the hands or arms.

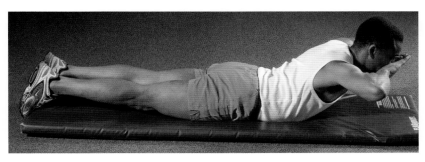

- Keep the toes in contact with the floor. The legs and hips do not move. Minimize all forward-to-backward and side-to-side movement.
- Lift the upper body to extend (arch) the low back until the upper chest is off of the mat (see photo).

Back extension.

Downward Movement

- Allow the upper body to lower slowly and under control back to the starting position.
- Maintain the same lower-body position with the back of the hands in contact with the face.

Simple Crunch or Pelvic Tilt

Adapted, by permission, from National Strength and Conditioning Association, 2008, *Exercise technique manual for resistance training,* 2nd Ed. (Champaign, IL: Human Kinetics), 165.

Following are the steps for the simple crunch or pelvic tilt.

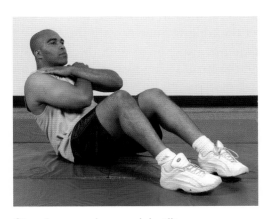

Starting Position

- Lie on your back on a floor mat.
- Flex the knees and hips to place the feet flat on the mat with the heels close to the buttocks.
- The thighs, knees, and feet should be next to each other.
- Fold the arms across the chest or abdomen.

Upward Movement

- Begin the exercise by flexing the neck to move the chin nearer to (but not touching) the upper chest and then curl the upper body to lift the upper back off the mat (see photo).

Simple crunch or pelvic tilt.

- Maintain the same lower-body position with the arms folded across the chest; do not lift the feet off the mat as the upper body is raised.
- Continue to curl the upper body toward the thighs until the upper back is off the mat and the elbows point toward the thighs. Be sure to use your abdominal muscles to curl your body upward.

Downward Movement

- Uncurl the upper body, then extend the neck slowly and under control back to the starting position; do not lift the buttocks off the floor.
- Maintain the same lower-body position, with the arms folded across the chest.

Lower-Body Exercises

Two simple exercises for upper and lower legs training are the lunge and the calf raise.

Lunge

Adapted, by permission, from National Strength and Conditioning Association, 2008, *Exercise technique manual for resistance training,* 2nd Ed. (Champaign, IL: Human Kinetics), 41-44.

Following are the steps for the lunge.

Starting Position

Place the feet hip-width apart with the toes pointing forward and hands on the hips.

Forward Movement

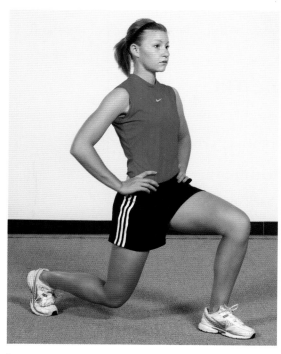

Lunge.

- Begin the exercise by taking one large step directly forward with one leg; this leg is called the lead leg.
- Keep the upper body erect and arms tight as the lead foot moves forward and contacts the floor. The trailing foot remains in its starting position, but as the lead leg steps forward, balance shifts to the ball of the trailing foot and the trailing knee flexes slightly.
- Plant the lead foot flat on the floor with the toes pointing forward.
- Once balance has shifted to both feet, flex the lead knee to lower the trailing knee toward the floor.
- The upper body must stay erect with the shoulders held back and the head facing forward. Sit back on the trailing leg; do not lean forward or look down.
- The lowest ideal body position is with the trailing knee 1 to 2 inches (3 to 5 cm) away from the floor, the lead knee flexed at a right angle, the lead lower leg at a right angle to the floor, and the lead foot flat on the floor (see photo). The lead knee must not extend past the toes of the lead foot.

Backward Movement

- Shift the balance forward to the lead foot and forcefully push off the floor with the lead foot. Do not jerk the upper body back; maintain its erect position.
- As the lead foot moves back toward the trailing foot, balance will shift back to the trailing foot. This will cause the heel of the trailing foot to regain contact with the floor.
- Carry the lead foot back to place it next to the trailing foot.
- As the lead foot is placed flat on the floor in its starting position, evenly divide the body's weight over both feet.
- Stand in the starting position, pause to gain full balance, then alternate lead legs and repeat the movement.

Calf Raise

Adapted, by permission, from National Strength and Conditioning Association, 2008, *Exercise technique manual for resistance training*, 2nd Ed. (Champaign, IL: Human Kinetics), 60-61.

Following are the steps for the calf raise:

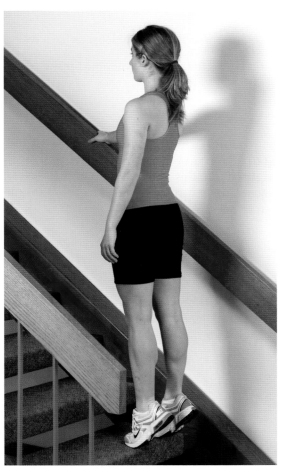

Calf raise.

Starting Position

- Place the balls of the feet on the nearest edge of the step with the legs and feet hip-width apart and parallel to each other. Reposition the body so the hips are under the shoulders and the knees are fully extended but not locked.
- Slowly allow the heels to lower fully under control to a comfortable, stretched position.

Upward Movement

- Begin the exercise by flexing the ankles slowly and under control.
- Keep the torso straight and the legs and feet parallel to each other.
- Apply even pressure on all toes; do not rise up only on the big or little toes.
- Do not push or swing the hips forward to help raise the weight.
- Continue the upward movement phase until the calf muscles are fully tightened (that is, the ankles are fully flexed; see photo).

Downward Movement

- Allow the heels to lower slowly and under control back to the starting position.
- At the bottom of the movement, do not bounce.

Resistance bands are an easy and completely portable option for strength training. So are everyday activities that involve carrying heavy loads, such as heavy gardening or carrying bags of groceries upstairs. Some aerobics classes use hand weights, which help give muscles an additional workout.

A few simple tips can help you get the most out of muscle-strengthening activities:

- Gradually increase the amount of resistance activity over a few weeks. Begin doing muscle-strengthening activities just one day a week. When you're comfortable with that amount, progress to two days a week. Over time, also increase the level of intensity until it becomes moderate to high.
- Effective muscle-strengthening activities should make muscles do more work than they are used to doing. Exercises should be repeated until it's difficult to do another repetition.
- Try to exercise all the major muscle groups of the body: the legs, hips, back, chest, abdomen, shoulders, and arms.
- Set a goal of doing muscle-strengthening activities at least twice a week.

 There is more information and resources on strength training available on the ALED Online Web site.

Avoiding Injuries

Nothing can sidetrack your physical activity efforts faster than an injury. One leading cause of activity-related injuries is trying to do too much, too fast. The best bet is to take a gradual approach. This helps strengthen muscles and stretch tendons slowly. Many people like to stretch as a way to warm up before activities. For a few simple stretching exercises, check pages 73-74 in chapter 6.

Activity Alert

How Far Have You Come?

 With this chapter, you've begun the second half of the program. It's a good time to take stock of your progress. Take a few minutes to look at the Assessing My Stage of Change questionnaire. Be honest. You can also download a copy of this form from the ALED Online Web site.

Assessing My Stage of Change

Goal: To do physical activity or exercise regularly, such as accumulating
- 150 min of moderate physical activity per week, or
- 75 min of vigorous physical activity per week, or
- a combination of moderate and vigorous physical activity each week, such as
  - a. 75 min of moderate and 40 min of vigorous physical activity, or
  - b. 90 min of moderate and 25 min of vigorous physical activity.

Moderate-Intensity Activity Examples
- Brisk walking
- Biking <10 mph (16 kph)
- Ballroom dancing
- General gardening, such as weeding
- Golfing (no cart)
- Any other physical activity where the exertion is similar to these

Vigorous-Intensity Activity Examples
- Jogging, running
- Tennis
- Biking >10 mph (16 kph)
- Aerobic dancing
- Heavy gardening, such as digging
- Any other physical activity where the exertion is similar to these

Regular physical activity means meeting or exceeding the physical activity goal described above.

For each statement, please mark *yes* or *no*.

1. I am currently physically active (at least 30 minutes per week). ❑ Yes ❑ No
2. I intend to become more physically active in the next 6 months. ❑ Yes ❑ No
3. I currently engage in **regular** physical activity. ❑ Yes ❑ No
4. I have been **regularly** physically active for the past 6 months. ❑ Yes ❑ No

Scoring Key
- *No* to 1, 2, 3, and 4 = **Precontemplation** stage
- *No* to 1, 3, and 4, *Yes* to 2 = **Contemplation** stage
- *Yes* to 1 and 2, *No* to 3 and 4 = **Preparation** stage
- *Yes* to 1 and 3, *Yes* or *No* to 2, *No* to 4 = **Action** stage
- *Yes* to 1, 3, and 4, *Yes* or *No* to 2 = **Maintenance** stage

From S.N. Blair, A.L. Dunn, B.H. Marcus, R.A. Carpenter, and P. Jaret, 2011, *Active Living Every Day*, 2nd ed. (Champaign, IL: Human Kinetics). Adapted from B.H. Marcus and L.R. Simkin, 1993, "The stages of exercise behavior," *Journal of Sports Medicine and Physical Fitness* 33: 83-88. By permission of B.H. Marcus.

What stage are you in now? If you've taken a step forward in the stages of change, congratulations! If not, don't fret. Even if you're thinking about activity more than you were, you're moving in the right direction. For tips on moving forward, take a look at appendix B. You'll find lots of good advice for each stage of change.

Progress toward any goal can require taking two steps forward and one step back. As long as you hold to your commitment and remind yourself why being physically active matters to you, you're still in the game. Before you start the next session, take a few minutes to write down three things that could help you take the next step. Your list might look something like this:

1. **Finding a convenient place where I feel safe walking at night**

2. **Asking people to support me**

3. **Getting myself motivated**

After you've made your list, brainstorm ways to get what you need. Check out local shopping malls that are open at night, for example. They can be a great place to walk. Consider rearranging your schedule to walk for 30 minutes in the morning. Tell friends and family about your plans, and ask them to give you their support and encouragement. To get motivated, revisit your checklist of all the benefits of physical activity on page 27.

In the next session, you'll learn more about using a step counter. Many people find these little devices to be useful motivational tools. Some of the participants in our programs say step counters are like having a personal coach with them every day, urging them to do a little more activity.

CHAPTER CHECKLIST

Before you move on to the next week's activities, make sure you've done the following:

- Learned to recognize all-or-nothing thinking
- Brainstormed ways around high-risk situations
- Identified your high-risk situations
- Tried out a few strength-training activities
- Completed the Assessing My Stage of Change questionnaire

 Checked out chapter 7 on the ALED Online Web site for more helpful resources and information for this chapter

References

Bennett, G.G., L.H. McNeile, K.Y. Wolin, D.T. Duncan, E. Puleo, and K.M. Emmons. 2007. Safe to walk? Neighborhood safety and physical activity among public housing residents. *Public Library of Science Medicine* 4(10): 1599-1606.

Department of Health and Human Services. 2008. *Physical activity guidelines for Americans.* Washington, DC: Government Printing Office.

Paterson, D.H., G.R. Jones, and C.L. Rice, 2007, Ageing and physical activity: evidence to develop exercise recommendations for older adults. *Canadian Journal of Public Health* 98 (Suppl 2): S69-108.

Portegjis, E. T. Rantanen, S. Sipila, P. Laukkanen, E. Hejkkinen. 2007. Physical activity compensates for increased mortality risk among older people with poor muscle strength. *Scandinavian Journal of Medicine and Science in Sports* 17(5): 473-9.

Simkin-Silverman, L.R., R.R. Wing, M.A. Boraz, and L.H. Kuller. 2003. Lifestyle intervention can prevent weight gain during menopause: Results from a 5-year randomized clinical trial. *Annals of Behavioral Medicine* 26(3): 212-220.

Thune, I. 1996. Physical activity and risk of colorectal cancer in men and women. *British Journal of Cancer* 73(9): 1134-1140.

Yanovski, J.A., S.Z. Yanovski, K.N. Sovik, T.T. Nguyen, P.M. O'Neil, and N.G. Sebring. 2000. A prospective study of holiday weight gain. *New England Journal of Medicine* 342(12): 861-867.

Chapter Eight

Step by Step

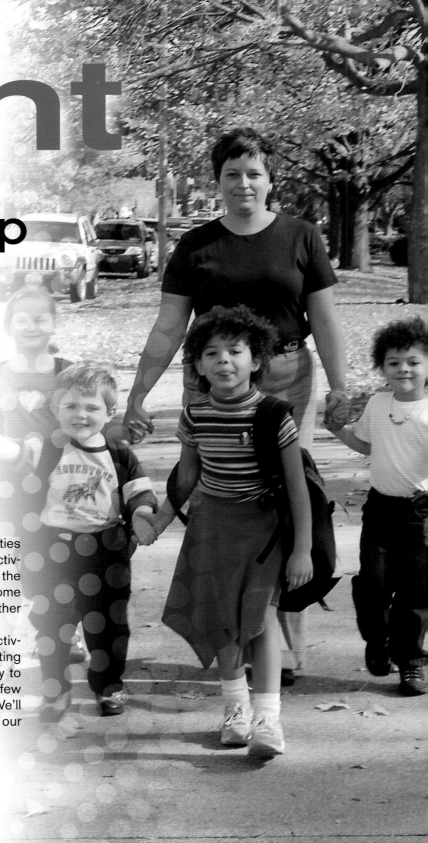

In This Chapter

- Reviewing ways to monitor activity
- Introducing the step counter
- Keeping a weekly activity log
- Resetting goals and rewards

By now we hope you've found plenty of opportunities to be active every day. Maybe you're feeling that activity is a natural part of your life. Hopefully, using the stairs instead of stepping on the elevator has become second nature. Walking to town to do errands rather than driving may be part of your routine.

There's only one drawback to a lifestyle activity program like ALED. When you're accumulating everyday activity in small chunks, it can be tricky to track your progress. In this chapter we'll look at a few familiar ways of monitoring your activity level. We'll also introduce a method that many participants in our programs liked best of all: the step counter.

Why Monitor?

We don't need to tell you that making a lasting change in your life can be hard. Some weeks you meet your goals; others you might fall short. It's easy to get discouraged if you're only looking at the small picture. By tracking your activity level each week, you see the big picture. You recognize where you have made progress and what helped you get there. You can also look back over a rocky period and understand the obstacles that got in your way. Tracking is a great way to stay motivated. It also provides a useful daily reality check.

Ways to Track Your Activity

By now you've tried a variety of ways to monitor your activity. One approach is to add up the time you spend doing physical activities. That method works well if your goal is to do at least 150 minutes of activity every week. Another way to monitor activity is to calculate the number of calories you burn while exercising. That approach is gratifying if your goal is not only to add activity but also to manage your weight.

In our studies, we introduced participants to a third way of measuring activity—step counters, or pedometers. We were surprised how popular they proved to be. Step counters are little gadgets that can be attached to your belt or waistband; some can be put in your pocket. They contain a mechanical pendulum that records every step you take. They're a great way to keep track of how much activity you do every day. They can also help you set goals for doing even more. Many participants told us that step counters are great motivators.

We're not the only fans of these cool little devices. Many findings show that step counters help motivate people to walk more. In 2007, a team at Stanford University reported findings from an analysis of 26 pedometer studies that included a total of 2,767 participants (Bravata et al. 2007). People who strapped on the devices averaged about 2,200 extra steps per day (1,800-2,200 steps equal 1 mi [1.6 km] depending on your speed and stride length). Pedometer users lost weight and lowered their blood pressure by an average of almost 4 points.

In another study (Schneider et al. 2006), this one with 56 overweight or obese volunteers who used pedometers, walkers who hit the goal of taking 10,000 steps a day lowered their body weight, lost body fat, slimmed down their waists and hips, and improved their cholesterol numbers. In general, the more steps people took, the more health benefits they enjoyed.

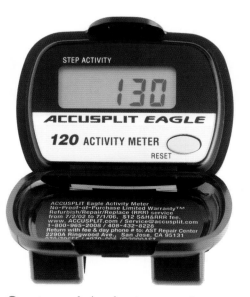

One type of simple step counter.

? Did You Know?

10,000 Steps Ghent

In Ghent, Belgium, a city-wide program called *10,000 Steps Ghent* offered free pedometers to encourage people to walk more (DeCocker, DeBourdeaudhuij, Brown, and Cardon 2007). Users of the devices added 896 steps to their average tally. Those extra steps meant an additional 8 percent of the participants reached the goal of 10,000 steps.

Selecting a Step Counter

If you took our advice in chapter 5, you should already have a step counter. If not, you can easily find a good one at your local sport store or online. For information, turn to page 56.

How to Use Your Step Counter

Follow these three simple steps when introducing step counter use into your daily routine.

Step 1: Wear it properly.

Step counters contain a small pendulum that moves each time you step. For the greatest accuracy, keep your step counter centered on your waistband or belt over your right or left hip bone. This should line up where the front crease of your trousers would be. Note that some step counters work in your pocket. Read the manufacturer's guide for proper placement and use.

Attach the step counter to your belt or waistband, centered over your right or left hip bone.

The step counter must be firmly attached. The best bet is to wear it on a belt. Another option is to attach it to the waistband of shorts, pantyhose, or underwear.

If you wear the step counter on your underwear or pantyhose, put the step counter inside the band of your garment, not outside. Be sure to remove it before you use the toilet—otherwise you might need to go fishing. We have discovered that even if step counters get wet, they still work once they dry out! Hopefully, you have a step counter that has a leash. This will also help prevent you from losing your step counter.

Step 2: Test it.

Good quality step counters are accurate and reliable. However, it is a good idea to put your step counter through a test.

1. Place the step counter at your waist as described previously.
2. Set the counter to zero by pressing the reset button. Close the cover.
3. Walk 50 steps, counting the steps in your head.
4. Open the display while it is still on your waistband to see how many steps the step counter registered. The number should be within 47 to 53 steps. If it is off by more than that, move the step counter slightly toward your belly button or your side and try the 50-step test again.
5. It may take a few trials to find the positioning that is right for your body. Because we are all built a little differently, the positioning of the counter may be slightly different from person to person. If the count is still off after several trials, return the step counter to the manufacturer for a replacement.

Step 3: Use it.

The purpose of using a step counter is to capture all your movement all day long.

- Put it on the first thing in the morning.
- Wear it all day, not just when you are exercising.
- If you change your clothing during the day, remember to reattach the step counter.
- Check the step counter several times a day to find out how close you are getting to your daily step goal.
- Record your daily steps right before you go to bed.

Did You Know?

When some 5,000 volunteers with type 2 diabetes set out to lose weight in a study called *Look AHEAD* (Action for Health in Diabetes), physical activity proved to be the most important determinant of success (Wadden et al. 2009). Researchers at the University of Pennsylvania School of Medicine reported that participants in the program lost 8.6 percent of their weight over the first year. They averaged 136 minutes of activity every week. Although the program included both healthy diet advice and exercise, physical activity proved to be the most important factor in long-term weight loss.

Activity Alert

Establish Your Starting Line

You already know from chapter 4 that goal setting is a key to successful behavior change. Setting physical activity goals using a step counter is easy. But you first have to know what your baseline step count is. Here's how to find it:

1. **Wear your step counter every day for a week, following the steps described previously. Keep track of your steps.**

2. **Use the Weekly Activity Log on page 99 to record your daily steps. You can download a copy of this form from the ALED Online Web site.**

3. **At the end of the week, calculate your average steps per day.**

4. **Set a reasonable daily goal to increase the average number of steps you take. If you averaged 4,000 steps a day, set a goal of 4,500 for the next week. Once you get there, raise the bar again. The ultimate goal should be about 10,000 steps each day. Our research shows that if you accumulate this many steps every day, you're most likely getting many benefits of physical activity. If you are trying to lose weight, you will need to do more, say 12,000 to 15,000 steps a day.**

Did You Know?

- Walking for 30 minutes at a brisk pace equals approximately 3,000 to 4,000 steps.
- Walking briskly during the four minutes of commercials between shows can tally up approximately 350 to 400 steps. How many steps can you take during commercials for your favorite TV program? Your overall goal should be to take 10,000 or more steps a day.

Setting Specific Goals

Now that you have learned how a step counter can help you set physical activity goals, it is a good time to step back and take a look at the long- and short-term goals you set in chapter 4. Look back to page 36. Have you attained your goals? Have you rewarded yourself as planned?

Step by Step: Weekly Activity Log

Week: _____

Day of week	Date	Actual steps	Notes
Monday			
Tuesday			
Wednesday			
Thursday			
Friday			
Saturday			
Sunday			
Total steps for week			
Average steps per day			

Week: _____

Day of week	Date	Actual steps	Notes
Monday			
Tuesday			
Wednesday			
Thursday			
Friday			
Saturday			
Sunday			
Total steps for week			
Average steps per day			

From S.N. Blair, A.L. Dunn, B.H. Marcus, R.A. Carpenter, and P. Jaret, 2011, *Active Living Every Day*, 2nd ed. (Champaign, IL: Human Kinetics).

If you haven't reached one or more of your goals, answer these questions:

- Was this a goal I really wanted for myself?
- Given what I now know, was the goal realistic?
- Did I do a good job specifying exactly what I was going to accomplish and by when?
- Did I have a way to track my progress toward the goal?

If you answered "no" to any of these questions, the problem may be how you set your goal. Go back to pages 34-36 to review the keys to successful goal setting. Then use the following space to revise and reset new goals and rewards for the second half of *Active Living Every Day*. Remember, your goals should be specific, personal, realis-

My Goals

A long-term goal I plan to achieve by _____ (date) is

_____

_____

_____

How I plan to monitor my progress

_____

_____

_____

Short-term goals that will help me reach my long-term goal

1. _____
2. _____
3. _____

1. How I plan to monitor my progress

_____

_____

_____

2. How I plan to monitor my progress

_____

_____

_____

3. How I plan to monitor my progress

_____

_____

_____

From S.N. Blair, A.L. Dunn, B.H. Marcus, R.A. Carpenter, and P. Jaret, 2011, *Active Living Every Day*, 2nd ed. (Champaign, IL: Human Kinetics).

tic, and measurable. You can set physical activity goals for minutes, miles, and now steps! You can also download a copy of this form from the ALED Online Web site.

Tracking Success

Setting goals and tracking success go hand in hand. You have seen how a step counter is a goal-setting tool. It is also a great way to monitor your progress. Our studies have found that participants who set specific goals and then keep track of their activity are the most successful at improving their overall fitness, losing weight, and decreasing their blood pressure.

Following is a tracking log that will help you track steps, minutes of activity, or both. An extra copy is included in appendix D on page 168. Make a few photocopies of that page, so you'll have plenty of activity logs.

My Tracking Log

Week: _____

Daily step goal: _____ **Reward:** _____

Minutes-of-activity goal: _____ **Reward:** _____

Other goals: _____ **Reward:** _____

Day of week	Date	Step goal	Actual steps	Minutes of activity		Notes
				Moderate	Vigorous	
Monday						
Tuesday						
Wednesday						
Thursday						
Friday						
Saturday						
Sunday						

From S.N. Blair, A.L. Dunn, B.H. Marcus, R.A. Carpenter, and P. Jaret, 2011, *Active Living Every Day*, 2nd ed. (Champaign, IL: Human Kinetics).

Weighing In

Don't Be Pound Foolish

Setting out to lose weight is fine. But a goal of losing a set number of pounds in a relatively short time can mean trouble. For starters, it's easy to get discouraged. When the pounds don't fall off over a few weeks, many people give up. It's important to remember that when you become active, you increase the amount of muscle mass in your body. So even if your weight on the scale remains the same, healthy changes are taking place.

Our studies have shown that even when people don't lose weight, increasing physical activity results in important health benefits, such as losing body fat and lowering both blood pressure and cholesterol levels. We looked specifically at whether being physically fit protected overweight men from dying prematurely (Lee, Blair, and Jackson 1999). We found that men who were obese but fit had a much lower risk of dying prematurely than obese men who were unfit. To our surprise, we found that obese, fit men had a lower risk of dying prematurely than even the lean but unfit men! The same association is true for women. If you want to lose weight, fine. Just make sure that's not your only goal. There are plenty of other excellent benefits you get from becoming physically active.

Losing Weight Takes Time

- The more active you are, the more muscle mass you develop.
- By increasing muscle mass, you increase your strength and fitness.
- Physical activity may reduce body fat, lower blood pressure, and lower cholesterol levels.
- Getting fit is as important as weight loss, maybe even more so.
- Make physical activity, not losing weight, your first priority.

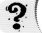 ## Did You Know?

Stepping Up the Intensity

How briskly do you need to walk in order to meet the criteria for moderate activity? In a 2009 study at San Diego State University, researchers studied 97 adults on exercise treadmills, measuring their energy expenditure while they walked (Marshall et al. 2009). They found that a moderate-intensity walking pace equals about 1,000 steps in 10 minutes. One way to meet the 2008 Physical Activity Guidelines for Americans (Department of Health and Human Services 2008), in other words, is to walk a minimum of 3,000 steps in 30 minutes on five days of the week.

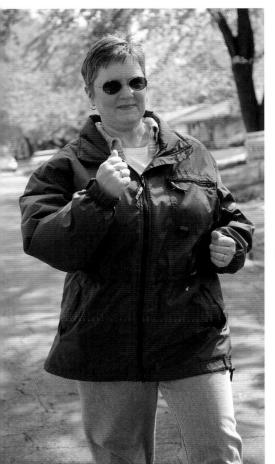

Electronic Coach

Wouldn't it be great to have a personal coach—someone to tell you how you're doing and encourage you when you slump? Step counters can be the next best thing.

From time to time during the day, check to see how many steps you've taken. If it's already midafternoon and you've tallied only 1,500 steps, it's time to get moving. Take an active coffee break, or get off the bus a few stops early and walk the rest of the way home. Go to the restroom four floors up or down instead of using the one on your floor. Use your step counter to monitor your progress during the day and to encourage you to push a little harder than yesterday. The one-day record for a participant in Project *Active* was 36,000 steps!

 ## Real Life

As hard as she tried, Jeannine never seemed to be able to stick with the program. Adding up the minutes spent climbing stairs or walking across the parking lot seemed too complicated to her. Setting aside the same time for a 15-minute walk every day didn't work, either. Never knowing whether she'd met her goal, she began to feel discouraged.

Then she tried a step counter. The first day out, she was thrilled to discover that the few changes she'd already made added up to

6,000 steps a day. Encouraged, she decided to add 1,000 steps more. Before work, she and her husband walked until she'd reached 1,000 steps. Added to her 6,000 steps from her daily activities, she reached a new high of 7,000 steps. Before long, Jeannine was averaging 10,000 steps a day. She got her husband a step counter too, and they had fun competing to see who could tally up the most steps.

Soon the whole family got into the act. Their teenage sons wanted step counters, and they all began to post their totals on a magnetic calendar on the refrigerator. Whoever won got to pick a place for a dinner out on the weekend.

Need a Boost?

Having a hard time keeping up? You're not alone. Making a lasting change in your life takes time. Remind yourself that the benefits are worth the effort and resolve to take two steps forward. Here are some tips that may help:

- Make sure your expectations and goals are reasonable. Remember, Rome wasn't built in a day.
- Plan ahead for situations that may sabotage your efforts. Think of ways to deal with these obstacles before they knock you off track.
- Getting bored and activities becoming stale are two common reasons people lose interest in physical activity. If that's the way you feel, push yourself to try one or two new activities, or find a new setting for the activities you love.
- Choose how to reward yourself in a special way for meeting your next important goal.
- Don't feel guilty if you haven't met your goals. Guilt only makes the problem seem worse than it is. Instead of moping, go for a brisk 10-minute walk. Then plan ways to add at least 30 minutes of activity each day for the next three days.

This week, you've used a step counter to calculate how many steps you typically take each day. You may find that a step counter does more than just keep track of your activities. If you're like many participants in our programs, you'll also find that these nifty devices encourage you to push yourself a little harder than yesterday.

CHAPTER CHECKLIST

Before you move on to the next week's activities, make sure you've done the following:

- Learned to use your step counter
- Found your baseline average number of steps per day
- Set new goals and rewards

 Checked out chapter 8 on the ALED Online Web site for more helpful resources and information for this chapter

References

Bravata, D.M., C. Smith-Spangler, V. Sundaram, A.L. Gienger, N. Lin, R. Lewis, C.D. Stave, I. Olkin, and J.R. Sirard. 2007. Using pedometers to increase physical activity and improve health: a systematic review. *Journal of American Medical Association* 298(19): 2296-2304.

DeCocker, K.A., I.M. DeBourdeaudhuij, W.J. Brown, and G.M. Cardon. 2007. Effects of 10,000 Steps Ghent: a whole-community intervention. *American Journal of Preventive Medicine* 33(6): 455-463.

Department of Health and Human Services. 2008. *Physical activity guidelines for Americans*. Washington, DC: Government Printing Office.

Lee, D.L., S.N. Blair, and A.S. Jackson. 1999. Cardiorespiratory fitness, body composition, and all-cause and cardiovascular disease mortality in men. *American Journal of Clinical Nutrition* 69(30): 373-380.

Marshall, S.J., S.S. Levy, C.E. Tudor-Locke, F.W. Kolkhorst, K.M. Wooten, M. Ji, C.A. Macera, and B.E. Ainsworth. 2009. Translating physical activity recommendations into a pedometer-based step goal: 3,000 steps in 30 minutes. *American Journal of Preventive Medicine* 36(5): 410-415.

Schneider, P.L., D.R. Bassett Jr., D.L. Thompson, N.P. Pronk, and K.M. Bielak. 2006. Effects of a 10,000 steps per day goal in overweight adults. *American Journal of Health Promotion* 21(2): 85-89.

Wadden, T.A., D.S. West, R.H. Neiberg, R.R. Wing, D.H. Ryan, K.C. Johnson, J.P. Foreyt, J.O. Hill, D.L. Trence, and M.Z. Vitolins; Look AHEAD Research Group. 2009. One-year weight losses in the Look AHEAD study: factors associated with success. *Obesity* 17(4): 713-722.

Chapter

Nine

Defusing Stress

In This Chapter

- Learning about the risks of stress
- Identifying stressful situations
- Exploring four techniques to reduce stress
- Setting priorities
- Finding ways to better manage your time

We hope that by now you are overcoming barriers to physical activity and have been planning for high-risk situations. One of the biggest stumbling blocks many people face is stress. Since so many of us deal with stress in our everyday lives, finding ways to defuse it is essential—especially when we're trying to make a lasting change for the better in our lives. That's why we devote this chapter to the all-important subject of stress and how to manage it.

At the beginning of this program, we asked you to close the book and take a walk. Now we're going to ask you to do something else you won't often see in a book about physical activity. Sit down, close your eyes, and take a deep breath. Fill your lungs with air from top to bottom. Draw the air in slowly. Let it out just as slowly. Then take another deep breath and let it out.

Go ahead and give it a try now.

Odds are good you feel calmer and more relaxed than before you paused to breathe. No matter how frazzled you feel, taking a deep breath can help relieve tension. That's why breathing exercises are an important part of many stress-reduction techniques, such as meditation and yoga.

The Big Deal About Stress

Why worry about stress in a book about physical activity? There is one simple reason. High levels of stress can wreak havoc with your motivation. People who are trying to give up smoking often falter during times of high stress. It weakens their willpower and makes it easier to reach for a cigarette.

Stress can also get in your way when you're trying to fit in at least 150 minutes of physical activity throughout the week. When a period of high stress comes along, you may find yourself feeling distracted or discouraged—unless you find ways to let off some steam.

We usually associate stress with negative events such as financial problems, marital difficulties, a rough phase at work, or being sick. But stress can also occur during the good times. Getting engaged, having a child, buying a new car, and looking for a new place to live are all stressful experiences.

Not all stress is the same. Sometimes stressful events arise suddenly and are over relatively quickly. Examples of acute stress include having a flat tire or breaking a favorite bowl or pitcher. It happens. We're upset. And then it's over. Unfortunately, some kinds of stress drag on for days and weeks on end. Examples of chronic stress include an unhappy relationship, trouble with our kids, or an unpleasant boss. Chronic stress has the most damaging effects on the body and mind.

Did You Know?

Why do so many people have trouble quitting smoking? One reason, for women especially, is that they gain weight when they kick the habit. As soon as those pounds show up on the bathroom scale, they reach for a cigarette! Being physically active can help quitters succeed. Researchers at Brown University found that women who exercised vigorously while trying to quit smoking were twice as likely to successfully quit smoking. One reason may be that exercisers gained half as much weight as their peers who did not participate in the exercise program. If you smoke, we encourage you to quit—when you're ready, of course. You're likely to find that being active helps you succeed (Marcus et al. 1999).

Fight or Flight

All of us have experienced the symptoms of acute stress in response to a feeling of danger. We get startled by a loud, unexpected noise or suddenly feel threatened by someone approaching on the street. Our hearts start pounding. Our blood pressure jumps. Our perception narrows to a sharp focus. We may even break into a sweat. Confronted with danger, our bodies are preparing for fight or flight. The fight-or-flight reaction no doubt saved our ancestors' lives when a wild animal suddenly threatened them. Even now the response may be a lifesaver. If you have to get out of the way of a speeding car, for instance, it's important to move quickly.

However, for most stressful situations we face today—a traffic jam, financial problems, or a confrontation with a coworker—the fight-or-flight response isn't appropriate. We're not going to haul off and punch that coworker, and we aren't likely to run away. Still, the surge of adrenaline and the sharp rise in blood pressure occurs. If it occurs again and again, it can strain mind and body, using energy and leading to nervous tension, sleeplessness, lowered immunity, and susceptibility to conditions such as high blood pressure, migraine or tension headaches, and depression.

Activity Alert

Stress Test

Are you under stress? Part of the answer depends on the pressures you feel at work and at home, but part of the answer also has to do with how you respond to those pressures. On this page are six questions that will help you gauge whether you deal with stress in a healthy or potentially unhealthy way. Imagine how you would react in these hypothetical situations.

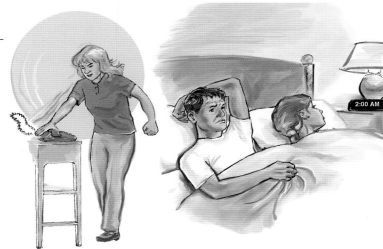

1. The cable repair company promised to arrive between 1:00 and 3:00, and it is almost 4:00. You've called twice, only to get a recorded message. You can feel your anger rising and your heart beating faster.	**True**	**False**
2. You have expensive tickets to a big game, and you're already running a little late. Your spouse is lingering over what coat to wear, though you've insisted twice that it's time to go. Suddenly you lose your patience and get angry.	**True**	**False**
3. Things are a little shaky at work, and now you've been asked to come in for a meeting with your supervisor on Friday. You know you shouldn't let it get to you. Still, you can't help but be anxious. For the next two nights, you find yourself waking up with a feeling of dread.	**True**	**False**
4. You've waited almost half an hour for a table at a restaurant, and suddenly the host seems to be seating a party that arrived after yours. You feel your face burn and your muscles tense up with anger.	**True**	**False**
5. In the middle of a phone conversation, a friend gets another call and puts you on hold. Thirty seconds pass. With your anger mounting, you slam down the phone.	**True**	**False**
6. It's been a long, hectic day, and you know you should take some time to relax and unwind, but you can't seem to slow down. On the way home, another driver almost cuts you off by mistake. You blast the horn, and hold it down long enough to show how angry you are.	**True**	**False**

From S.N. Blair, A.L. Dunn, B.H. Marcus, R.A. Carpenter, and P. Jaret, 2011, *Active Living Every Day*, 2nd ed. (Champaign, IL: Human Kinetics).

In each hypothetical situation, there are multiple ways to respond when something goes wrong. You can get mad when a driver inadvertently cuts you off, or you can shrug it off, reminding yourself that you've done the same thing sometimes. You can slam down the phone when your friend puts you on hold, or you can wait until she gets back on the line and then gently say you'd rather have her call you back than put you on hold.

Look back over your answers. If you answered "true" to most questions, you may be what psychologists call a *hot reactor*. Instead of staying cool when problems arise, your heart rate accelerates, your muscles tense up, and you feel your anger surging. The more times you answered "true," the more important it is to find healthy ways to defuse stress. Regardless of your answers to the questions, most of us can use a few stress-busting strategies.

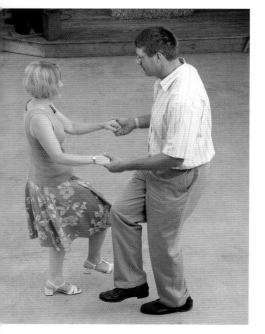

Coping With Stress

There are many ways to let off steam. Not all of them work for everyone. The important thing is to find a strategy that works well for you. Here are some great ways to cope.

Take a Walk—or a Swim or a Bike Ride

Walking, running, bicycling, swimming, dancing, and other physical activities are great ways to unwind and blow off steam. Physical activity also has other long-lasting benefits. Consistent moderate to vigorous physical activity, for example, can lower your heart rate (Murtagh et al. 2005). Studies of people who have lowered their heart rates have found that they have lower heart rate responses during and after mental stress compared with people who have not been consistently active (Dishman et al. 2002). Other studies of activity and stress show that stress hormone levels are lower during a bout of physical activity in people who are fit compared with those who are unfit (Nabkasorn et al. 2005). In addition to reducing the physical responses to stress, physical activity can improve mood and reduce symptoms of anxiety and depression (Department of Health and Human Services 2008).

Relax—One Body Part at a Time

Another helpful technique is called *progressive relaxation*, or deep muscle relaxation. Why concentrate on muscles? Muscles communicate with nerves, and nerves directly connect to the brain. By relaxing your muscles, you can calm your mind. To practice this technique, sit in a chair or lie on a bed, and start with your hands, tensing and relaxing each muscle group at least twice, while inhaling and exhaling deeply and slowly. Next, move to the muscles of your shoulders. Try the muscles in your face or wherever you can feel the tension build. As you become skilled at this, you'll be able to tense and relax your muscles and reduce stress quickly when it occurs. You can use this stress buster sitting at your desk or behind the wheel in a traffic jam.

Use Your Imagination

A technique called *guided imagery* can also help ease the mind. It's simple: Just imagine yourself in a setting where you are perfectly relaxed. It could be a mountain meadow with a stream bubbling past. Perhaps your favorite spot on earth is a beach with the surf whispering nearby or a garden with birds singing and the smell of roses. You choose. What's important is thinking of a restful, relaxing, supportive place. Try to involve all five senses. Imagine the feel of the sun on your face, the smells

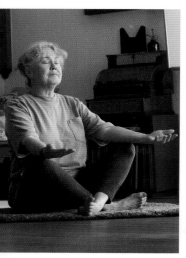

Dancing and relaxation can help ease stress.

carried on the breeze, the sounds of nature, the color of the leaves and flowers, or the taste of crisp, cool mountain stream water. As you feel your body beginning to relax, breathe deeply, inhaling and exhaling. Stay in your imaginary spot for 5 or 10 minutes, and you'll feel the tension of the day fade away.

Have a Laugh

Anything that makes you laugh also reduces stress. A good laugh relaxes muscles and stimulates the production of stress-relieving chemicals in the brain. Watch a favorite movie or television show that is usually good for a laugh, or schedule time to get together for conversation with friends you find entertaining.

Did You Know?

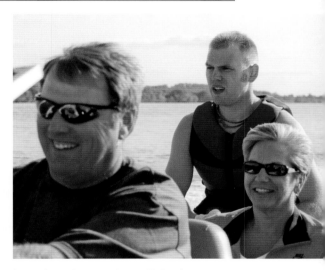

Laughter is good medicine. In a study led by physician Lee Berk at Loma Linda University (Berk et al. 1989), researchers studied the effect of viewing a 60-minute humorous video. Blood tests to measure biochemical changes in hormones associated with stress showed that the video watchers had improved levels of the hormones. These findings suggest that laughter may help reduce the harmful ways in which our body naturally responds to stress. Even anticipating a laugh—preparing to watch a funny film, for example—causes immune-boosting hormones to rise and stress hormones to fall. In Dr. Berk's latest study, laughing was associated with a 26 percent jump in levels of good cholesterol and a 66 percent drop in levels of C-reactive protein, a measure of inflammation linked to both heart disease and diabetes risk (Berk and Tan 2009). Berk jokingly calls watching funny videos *laughercise* because the benefits are so similar to those of physical activity.

Laughter is good medicine!

Real Life

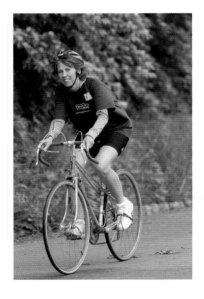

If type A people are high-pressure, hard-driven types, Rosa figured she must be type AAA. The owner of her own company, she worked long hours and had little patience for anything that got in her way. She didn't realize how stressed out she'd become until she had an accident driving home from the office one night. Annoyed at the heavy traffic, she'd been following the car ahead too closely. When the traffic ahead came to a sudden stop, she couldn't brake in time and rear-ended the car ahead of her.

That was it, Rosa decided. It was time to cool off. She bought a book about stress reduction and tried a few techniques. Given her driven nature, meditation and imagery felt to her as if she were wasting time. When she read that physical activity can relieve stress, she decided to give it a try. She could stand to lose a few pounds, and her doctor had been hounding her about getting exercise anyway. For half an hour at noon, she either walked or took her bike out for a spin on a nearby bike path. Gradually she began to notice that she wasn't getting as steamed up as she used to. The muscles in her back and shoulders no longer felt so tense. She also noticed that she was beginning to look forward to getting a little exercise over the noon hour just for the pleasure of it. She knew things were changing for the better when her employees got together and gave her a joke present for her birthday—handlebar streamers for her bike.

Stress-Busting Tips

We've already looked at some useful techniques to ease stress. Here are a few other ways to handle the pressures of daily life without turning yourself inside out:

- **Deal with the cause.** You may not be able to change the cause of your stress completely, but you can find ways to relax things a little. If a bad relationship with your neighbor is getting you down, consider one or two changes you could make to ease the situation. Sometimes all it takes is thinking about the situation differently.

- **Call on your support troops.** Talking with someone helps ease any kind of stress or strain. You may even get some good advice on how to deal with the problems or pressure you're experiencing.

- **Take care of yourself.** When you feel run down, situations often look worse than they are. Your ability to cope may be hindered. It's important to get enough sleep, eat a healthy diet with at least five servings of fruits and vegetables a day, and do something nice for yourself regularly.

- **Take one thing at a time.** Sometimes our lives are so crowded and hectic that we feel overwhelmed by the sheer number of demands on us. That's when it's important to stop, take a deep breath, and set realistic short-term goals. Put things that are most important to you at the top of the list. Take pride in what you accomplish. Be sure to give yourself a pat on the back now and then.

- **Learn to worry constructively.** It never pays to worry for the sake of worrying. Instead, think about constructive ways to deal with the stresses in your life. One approach that often helps is to think about the problem as if it were someone else's instead of your own. How would you advise that person? Then consider taking your own advice.

- **Accept things you cannot change.** There's nothing worse than banging your head against a wall that just won't move. Unfortunately, there are plenty of things in life we can't change, but we can change the way we think about them.

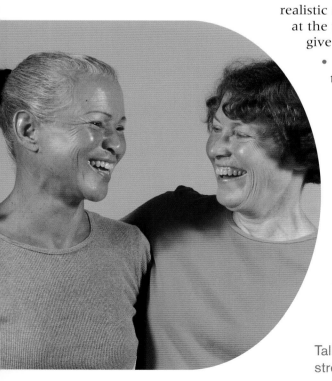

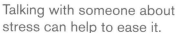

Talking with someone about stress can help to ease it.

Myth Busters

"All it really takes to change a bad habit is willpower."

Surprisingly, many psychologists say it's a bad idea to rely too much on willpower when you're trying to make a change for the better. Willpower turns out to be a limited resource. Sure, you can say no to that rich dessert at lunch easily enough. But if you have to resist the temptation of eating cookies during your midafternoon break and then resist eating chips when you go out for dinner, your willpower may run out. We can't deny ourselves again and again simply by relying on willpower. Even the strongest determination needs to be backed up by planning and specific strategies. In this example, you might make sure you have a healthy alternative to those cookies so that you can enjoy something during your break. And you may have a plan in place to tell the waiter at your favorite Mexican restaurant not to bring chips to the table or to bring only half a bowl. Having a few strategies to relieve stress can also help. Stress can quickly erode willpower.

Activity Alert

My Plan for Reducing Stress

Now it's time to try out some techniques for reducing stress. This week, experiment with at least two stress-busting techniques. Just to show you we mean business, we're going to ask you to put your plan in writing. Write down two ways of coping with stress that you'll try this week. For example, you might get some additional physical activity and try progressive muscle relaxation. Or you might rent a funny movie or try imagery. Be aware of how you're feeling before, during, and after you use each technique. You can also download a copy of this form from the ALED Online Web site.

Two stress-reducing techniques to try this week

1. _____

2. _____

How well did stress-reducing strategy 1 work? (Circle one.)

Very well   Moderately well   Not at all

How well did stress-reducing strategy 2 work? (Circle one.)

Very well   Moderately well   Not at all

From S.N. Blair, A.L. Dunn, B.H. Marcus, R.A. Carpenter, and P. Jaret, 2011, *Active Living Every Day*, 2nd ed. (Champaign, IL: Human Kinetics).

If these two techniques didn't help you let off steam, try another. If the strategies you tried worked moderately well, give yourself more time to practice them. Even relaxing doesn't always come easy. Some people have to practice a while before they get the hang of it.

If the techniques worked very well, congratulations. Now write down some situations when you plan to use the techniques (when work is hectic, for instance, or after a long day, when the kids are in bed and the house is finally quiet).

_____

_____

Did You Know?

Who's in Charge, Anyway?

Compared with people who feel frazzled when things get stressful, stress-hardy people seem to have three important attitudes, or the three Cs of surviving stress: challenge, commitment, and control. Stress-hardy people

- see change as a *challenge*, not a threat;
- feel a strong *commitment* to their jobs, their families, and their decision to change; and
- have a firm sense of *control* over their lives and how they spend their time.

The third C is one reason time management is so important. By gaining control over how you spend the time you have, you'll lower stress and increase self-confidence. You'll also feel at the end of the day that you've accomplished what really matters to you.

Managing Your Time

One of the biggest sources of stress is not having enough time to do what needs to be done. If you're like most people, you probably wish there were 36 hours in the day. Only then would you have time to do all the things you need and want to do.

Feeling pressed for time has another unfortunate consequence. It's one of the chief reasons people say they don't get enough physical activity.

Like it or not, we're stuck with 24 hours in the day. It's up to us to decide how to use that time. We can't do away with some demands in our lives, such as work and family responsibilities. However, we can manage them more wisely than we do. All of us, no matter how hectic our schedules are, have time we can spend in any way we choose.

Setting Priorities

The first step is to set priorities. What are the things you really value? What are the things you most want to accomplish? We mean *you*. Don't worry about other people's priorities for the moment. Concentrate on your own.

One handy way is to make a list of the things you do each day. Then rate the activities using a 4-point scale, with 1 being the things you value highly and 4 being things you don't value. Here's a sample priority list of activities:

1 Value highly	2 Value somewhat	3 Neutral	4 Don't value
Task		**Value**	
Checked the news online		3	
Taught classes		1	
Wrote report		2	
Walked at lunch		1	
Met with parents		1	
Played with children		1	
Cleaned house		3	
Watched television		4	
Talked to friends on phone		2	

A quick glance over those priorities makes it clear which activities matter and which don't. Anything that ranks a 4—watching television in this example—you can easily replace with something that matters more (such as getting out and walking for half an hour). You don't necessarily have to replace one task with another. You can borrow a little time from one to devote to another. In this case, you could decide to give up some of the time spent reading the paper to take a 15-minute walk after breakfast. Another option is to combine tasks. Turn time with friends into activity by suggesting walking together rather than talking on the telephone, for example.

Activity Alert

My Priorities

Take a few minutes to think about the tasks you did yesterday. Include everything that required 15 minutes or more of your time. Give each activity a value from 1 to 4. Be honest with yourself about the priority each activity has in your mind. The only activities that score a 1 should be those that really matter to you. You can also download a copy of this form from the ALED Online Web site.

What Matters?

1 Value highly	2 Value somewhat	3 Neutral	4 Don't value
Task			**Value**

From S.N. Blair, A.L. Dunn, B.H. Marcus, R.A. Carpenter, and P. Jaret, 2011, *Active Living Every Day*, 2nd ed. (Champaign, IL: Human Kinetics).

Look back at your list. If it consists primarily of 1s and 2s, you're doing the things that matter most to you and are managing your time well. If your list includes more 3s and 4s, you're doing things that you really don't value. You probably feel frustrated and stressed, and it's no wonder. Now's the time to work on ways to spend more time doing the things you value most. You'll be happier and less frustrated, and the people around you will probably be happier, too.

Setting Boundaries

Setting boundaries is easier said than done, of course. We are surrounded by people whom we depend on or who depend on us. If you have a family, for instance, your kids come first. If it's a question of helping one of them with his homework or taking a brisk walk after dinner, obviously you're going to help your child. If your wife is ill, you naturally want to help care for her. If you're going through a stressful time at work, it's hard not to let that stress spill over into your personal life.

But as important as other people are in your life, your own well-being and happiness also matter. You can't be a good parent or a good caregiver unless you're also taking care of yourself and doing things you value.

That's why it's so important to set boundaries. Boundaries mark off territory. They help you stay true to your priorities and your values. One example might be marking off a time that you reserve for yourself to accomplish the things that matter to you—7:00 to 7:30 in the evening, for instance, when you walk briskly around the neighborhood. You can also set boundaries by making up your mind that once you leave the office, you also leave the stresses of your working life behind.

Here's another example of how a boundary might help. Let's say your spouse is a little threatened by your efforts to become more active. It may be necessary to set up an emotional boundary and to clearly communicate that your exercise is important to you. In a sense, you put a fence around your efforts to be more active in order to protect them from being undermined by other people. By doing so, you'll give your plans time to grow and flourish, just as you might nourish a small garden.

Real Life

Marcus began each week full of good intentions. By midweek, though, he was skipping his walk over the noon hour because something else always came up. When he sat down to list all the things he needed and wanted to do, he realized how crowded his day was. With work, the kids, the house, and all the other demands on him, he didn't feel like he had much control over his schedule.

Looking at how he spent his time was a revelation for Marcus. He realized that not all the demands on his time were equally important, nor did he place the same value on them. Once the kids were in bed, Marcus and his wife had gotten into the habit of stretching out on the sofa and watching television. But there were only two programs Marcus really enjoyed. Also, it was often hard to get away over the lunch hour. If he made walking for half an hour a top priority, however, he realized he could usually do that and still get his work done.

Marcus changed his activity plan to make better use of his time. He set a goal of walking at least three days a week during the noon hour. That allowed for two days off whenever his schedule became too hectic. He and his wife agreed that on the other two nights of the week, instead of vegging on the sofa, they'd walk through the neighborhood together.

To his surprise, Marcus found that he had plenty of time to be active. The trick was making activity a top priority.

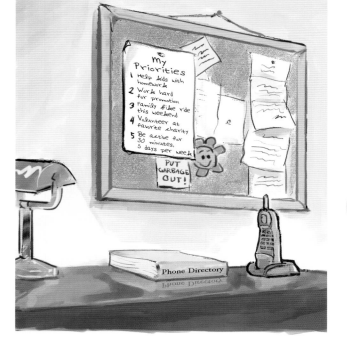

 ## Weighing In

Like most health experts, we're convinced that regular physical activity is a crucial component of any weight-loss plan and an even more important part of a plan to prevent weight gain. Just as important, of course, is controlling the number of calories you eat and drink. In virtually all studies, people who combine activity with a sensible eating

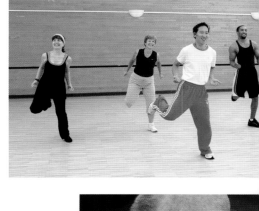

plan are more likely to maintain weight loss than those who simply diet. The typical weight loss is in the range of 5 to 10 pounds (2.3-4.5 kg). That may not sound like a lot, but it's enough to lower the risk of heart disease and diabetes as well as certain forms of cancer.

Not everyone who increases physical activity will lose weight. People who are lean to start with don't have much fat to lose. The people most likely to lose weight are those who have been inactive and are slightly overweight. Studies show that when people use dieting alone for weight loss, they regain most of the weight within a year or two. The best success in losing weight and keeping it off occurs in people who combine exercise with a sensible eating plan.

Just as important, physical activity helps prevent weight gain. In fact, the physical activity guidelines for Americans note that the strongest evidence for the health benefits of activity include prevention of weight gain (Department of Health and Human Services 2008). That's why efforts to encourage more active lifestyles among children and young adults are so important to a lifetime of good health. There's moderate to strong evidence that exercise helps prevent abdominal obesity—another crucial benefit. Activity also helps maintain muscle tissue when you're on a calorie-restricted diet. That's important to health and to how you look in the mirror.

Time-Management Techniques

Managing your stress level means managing your time well. People use a variety of techniques for managing time. One effective method is to list the activities that you plan to accomplish for the day. You can do this the night before or first thing in the morning. If you prefer to plan for an entire week, write up your to-do list on Sunday night or Monday morning.

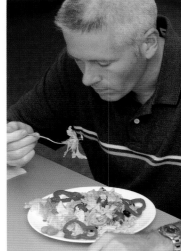

Exercising and eating right help keep the weight off.

Another approach is to use a calendar and assign your top-priority items a specific time during the day. That's especially important if you are more productive or energetic at one time of day than another. For example, some people wake up in the morning ready to go and are fully alert. Others do their best work in the afternoon or evening. Schedule your must-do tasks for your best part of the day.

Whatever approach you choose, be realistic. After all, there's only so much any of us can accomplish in a day. A list that is too ambitious will only make you frustrated and discouraged. Also, be sure to give yourself time for breaks. Physical activity can be a terrific break from desk work.

Finally, don't be discouraged if your best-laid plans get thrown off schedule. Sometimes unavoidable demands take up more time than you expected, squeezing out other tasks. At work, for instance, staff meetings often go longer than anticipated. At home, you may find that once you start tidying up the house, you discover many things that need your attention. If you see a time squeezer on the horizon, try to schedule it for later in the day, after you've done your top-priority items (which hopefully include physical activity).

"I Should" Versus "I Want To"

Take a moment to look back at your list of priorities. Many top items are probably things you know you should do. One reason most people try to increase their activity is they know they should, but *should* only goes so far. To make any lasting change, you have to turn what you should do into something you value doing. That way you're likely to find the time to do it.

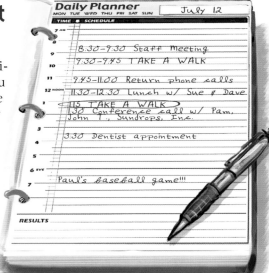

 ## Activity Alert

Of course, we have an ulterior motive in asking you to list your priorities. We're hoping that by now, getting at least 150 minutes of physical activity each week is right up there with the most important activities of your day. We'll even settle for second place on a day when you've got lots of other important things going on. However, if you honestly can't make activity a top priority in your day, you might want to look back to revisit the list of benefits you hope to get from being active.

Take a moment to think about tomorrow and the coming week. What do you have to do? What do you want to do? Use the following space to organize your tasks into three priority categories: must do, hope to do, and do if I have time. Make the list as complete as possible. Create a list just for tomorrow if that seems appropriate, or think about the entire week.

This Week's Priorities

Date _____

Must do_____

_____

_____

Hope to do _____

_____

_____

Do if I have time _____

_____

_____

From S.N. Blair, A.L. Dunn, B.H. Marcus, R.A. Carpenter, and P. Jaret, 2011, *Active Living Every Day*, 2nd ed. (Champaign, IL: Human Kinetics).

Where did you list physical activity? We hope it's a must-do item. Now carry this list with you wherever you go so you can easily remember your top priorities.

You may have noticed that we've been using the word *management* a lot, as in stress management and time management. We've talked about setting priorities and establishing boundaries. There's a good reason for that. Making a change in your life requires you to take charge—to manage the complicated parts of your life successfully. That's one of the hidden benefits of a program like this. Not only do people become more active, they also discover that they can take more control of their lives. They can arrange their time to get more pleasure out of life and to accomplish what they want. They can manage the inevitable stresses of everyday life and stay active and healthy.

In the next chapter, you'll use your newfound confidence and management skills to identify and add new opportunities for activity into your routine.

CHAPTER CHECKLIST

Before you move on to the next week's activities, make sure you've done the following:

- Identified ways to relax
- Made a plan for dealing with stress
- Assigned priorities to the things you need to do and want to do
- Organized the tasks for the coming week according to must do, hope to do, and do if I have time

 Checked out chapter 9 on the ALED Online Web site for more helpful resources and information for this chapter

References

Berk, L.S., and S.A. Tan. 2009. Mirthful laughter as adjunctive therapy in diabetes care increases HDL cholesterol and attenuates inflammatory cytokines and hs-CRP and possible CVD risk. Presented at the 122nd Annual Meeting of the American Physiological Society, New Orleans.

Berk, L.S., S.A. Tan, W.F. Fry, B.J. Napier, J.W. Lee, R.W. Hubbard, J.E. Lewis, and W.C. Eby. 1989. Neuroendocrine and stress hormone changes during mirthful laughter. *American Journal of Medicine and Science* 298(6): 390-396.

Department of Health and Human Services. 2008. *Physical activity guidelines for Americans.* Washington, DC: Government Printing Office.

Dishman, R.K., E.M. Jackson, and Y. Nakamura. 2002. Influence of fitness and gender on blood pressure responses during active or passive stress. *Psychophysiology* 39(5):568-76.

Marcus, B.H., A.E. Albrecht, T.K. King, A.F. Parisi, B. Pinto, M. Roberts, R.S. Niaura, and D.B. Abrams. 1999. The efficacy of exercise as an aid to smoking cessation in women: a randomized controlled trial. *Archives of Internal Medicine* 159(11): 1229-1234.

Murtagh, E.M., C.A. Boreham, A. Nevill, L.G. Hare, and M.H. Murphy. 2005. The effects of 60 minutes of brisk walking per week, accumulated in two different patterns, on cardiovascular risk. *Preventive Medicine* 41(1): 92-7.

Nabkasorn, C., N. Miyai, A. Sootmongkol, S. Junprasert, H. Yamamoto, M. Arita, et al. 2005. Effects of physical exercise on depression, neuroendocrine stress hormones and physiological fitness in adolescent females with depressive symptoms. *European Journal of Public Health J Public Health* 16(2): 179-84.

Chapter Ten

Finding New Opportunities to Be Active

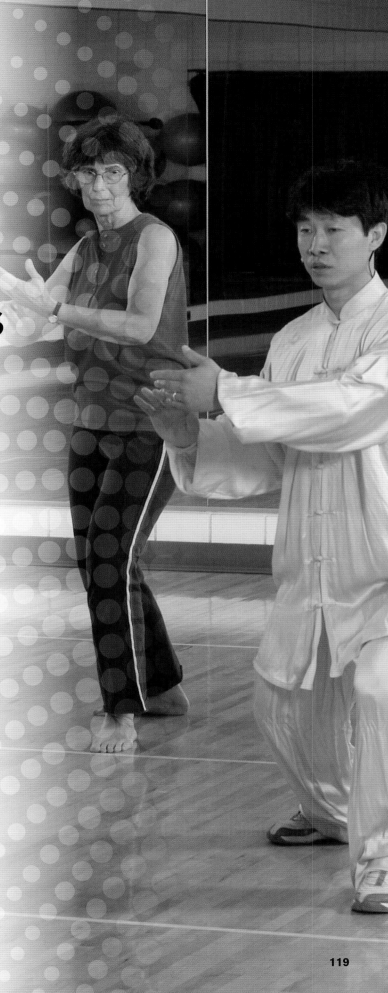

In This Chapter

- Identifying new ways to be physically active
- Checking out options for physical activity in your community
- Selecting in-home exercise equipment
- Adding a little extra activity to your weekly schedule

For almost all of our development as a species, we relied on physical activity to survive. As hunter-gatherers, we spent much of our days moving about and working hard to get enough to eat. Later we learned to grow crops by hand and build communities with sheer muscle power. Our bodies evolved and adapted for this kind of strenuous activity.

More recently, labor-saving devices have steadily diminished opportunities for physical activity. First came the wheel. Then came carriages and cars. Before long there were riding mowers and elevators and other devices that saved us from having to burn calories. Now with home-shopping TV channels and the Internet, we don't even need to get up from a chair to go shopping.

On top of that, we've created a world of unprecedented plenty. We enjoy a greater variety of foods than many people dreamed of in previous generations. Unfortunately, we're paying the price for our lack of physical activity and excessive eating in the form of obesity, heart disease, and other chronic diseases.

Becoming a Modern-Day Hunter-Gatherer

We can't go back to being hunter-gatherers. But to be healthy, we must find ways to resist the sedentary pressures of the modern world. Luckily, there are plenty of opportunities. You've probably already taken advantage of a few.

Alternative Ways to Become More Active

Instead of	Try
Hiring someone to do your yard work	Doing it yourself
Driving to the store for one item	Walking or riding your bike
Going to the movies on a Saturday afternoon	Going for a bike ride or hike
Taking a lazy vacation	Enjoying an active vacation
Taking the escalator or elevator	Climbing the stairs

Checking Out Community Resources

Most communities have a wealth of recreational opportunities. Some are sponsored by park and recreation departments. Sometimes people who enjoy bicycling, hiking, square dancing, or swimming form their own groups. Most of these groups welcome newcomers, even people with little or no experience. Examples include the following:

Cycling clubs

Dancing clubs

Fun runs and walks

Golfing leagues

Skating groups

Orienteering clubs

Outdoor clubs

Racquetball leagues

Rowing and canoeing clubs

Running clubs

Soccer leagues

Swimming clubs

Tennis leagues

Volleyball leagues

Basketball leagues

Walking clubs

Activity Alert

Searching for Activities

This week, check out what your community has to offer. There are many ways to get information.

- Learn about the activities provided by your local recreation center or the park and recreation department.
- Search your town or county Web site for other useful information.
- Scan the local newspaper for information on recreational activities.
- Visit the popular Internet site Yelp (www.yelp.com). It includes a category called *active life*, which offers insider tips on great local walking areas, swimming pools, and other opportunities to be active.
- Use Google, Bing, or another search engine to look for local recreational opportunities.

If you don't have Internet access at home, you can probably find it at your local library. Be sure to also check the ALED Online Web site for links to other resources.

You can also try the old-fashioned way, consulting a book at the library or bookstore. Many books have maps of local hiking and biking trails. Larger cities may have recreational guides that list a variety of activities. Sporting goods stores and bike shops are also useful sources of information. Make a point this week to seek out information. Use the form on page 122 to keep track of what you find. You can also download a copy of this form from the ALED Online Web site.

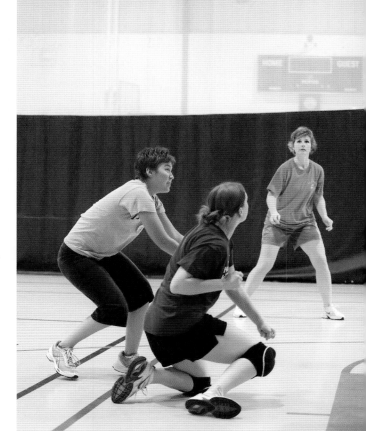

Park and recreation departments offer a wealth of activity opportunities, even for adults.

New Opportunities to Be Active

Share your list with friends and neighbors to see if they know of other resources. After you've made your list, circle your top two choices, and give them a try.

New Opportunities for Activity

Parks (local, state, national)	Location	Comments

Walking, biking, and hiking trails	Location	Comments

Recreation centers	Location	Comments

Activity clubs	Location	Comments

Dance halls or schools	Location	Comments

Other	Location	Comments

From S.N. Blair, A.L. Dunn, B.H. Marcus, R.A. Carpenter, and P. Jaret, 2011, *Active Living Every Day*, 2nd ed. (Champaign, IL: Human Kinetics).

Did You Know?

For years, scientists funded by the National Institutes of Health have been studying the Pima Indians in Arizona. Their goal is to help the Pimas fight a dangerous epidemic. Many Americans are overweight or obese, but the Pimas are at extreme risk. As many as 75 percent are obese, and many suffer from diabetes.

This is not true of all Pimas, however. Those who continue to till the land and carry water by hand in parts of Mexico remain lean and remarkably healthy. Virtually none of them has diabetes or obesity. Researchers suspect that the Pimas adapted to their harsh environment by evolving to make the energy of every calorie they ate go as far as it could. Those most likely to survive were those who had a so-called thrifty gene. When food was scarce, this gene kept people alive. Pima Indians in the United States are plagued by obesity because they get significantly less physical activity than the Pimas in Mexico (Esparz et al. 2000). They also have access to a much greater variety and amount of food.

The Pima Indians of Arizona and Mexico illustrate a problem many of us face. Our bodies were built for a different environment. In our current world, we have to work hard not to gain weight. All of us would be healthier if we could add more physical activity into our lives.

Real Life

Cheryl had tried bicycling, hiking, and in-line skating, but none of them gave her much pleasure. Then a friend invited her to attend a hip-hop dance class. Cheryl was amazed to see that the other participants were her age and a little older, not young kids as she had suspected. But boy, could they move, and they looked like they were having a great time. Cheryl decided to give it a try.

Joining the dance class came at just the right time in her life. She had recently divorced and was experiencing bouts of depression. Dancing, especially after work when she was uptight and weary, helped restore her spirits. She made friends with the other dancers, who all provided a welcome sense of camaraderie. She's now in the best physical shape of her life. Just as important, she's found a real passion.

Dance, Dance, Dance

If you haven't danced to your favorite music in years, now's the time to give it a whirl. Whether you prefer the Texas two-step, a stately waltz on the ballroom floor, or a lively salsa number, dancing is a wonderful way to relax and be active. It's great fun to dance with your kids or grandkids. Even dancing by yourself is a great way to unwind and get your heart rate up. Have some boring housework to do? Try putting on your favorite music and dancing while doing chores. Time will fly by and your house will be sparkling. If you want to get serious about dancing, check out the community listings for dance

Dancing is a great way to be active!

classes or dancing clubs. Or, challenge your kids or grandkids to a round or two of active video games such as *Dance Dance Revolution* or *Wii Fit*.

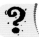

Did You Know?

A Tale of Two Lifestyles

Just how much less active are we today compared with people living three or four generations ago? A few years back, researchers used a unique study to answer that question. They asked 98 Old Order Amish men and women to wear step counters all day long for seven days. Old Order Amish don't use automobiles or modern electrical appliances. They still farm using animal-powered plows and implements. On average, the Amish men accumulated 18,425 daily steps, and the women accumulated 14,196 daily steps. By comparison, sedentary adults in the United States take about 5,000 steps per day. Not surprisingly, none of the Amish men was obese, and only 9 percent of the women were obese, compared with more than 33 percent of American men and 35 percent of women (Bassett, Schneider, and Huntington 2004).

Most of us can't live as the Amish do. We certainly can't spend our days on foot tracking down our food. But we can become hunter-gatherers of new ways to move more.

Selecting Home Exercise Equipment

Activity groups and hiking trails aren't for everyone. Some people prefer to be active in the privacy of their homes. That's great. There are plenty of advantages to home exercise equipment such as treadmills, stair-climbers, or rowing machines. First is convenience. Your own personal gym is there whenever you feel the urge to get up and moving. At-home equipment is terrific for rainy days or days when it's too hot or cold to go outside. Just having equipment in the house is a reminder to be active. You can set up your treadmill or stair machine in front of a television and watch your favorite show. After all, you don't have to be a couch potato to enjoy a little TV time. You can also read or listen to music. Over time, buying equipment can be cheaper than paying for a membership at a gym. Finally, several family members can use the exercise equipment. That's important because children who see their parents being active are likely to be active themselves.

There are some potential drawbacks, however. If your activity interests change, you'll be stuck with a piece of equipment you don't use. (You can always try to sell it on Craigslist or eBay, of course.) Unless you have the space to set up the equipment and leave it in place, it may spend more time in storage than in use. Exercise equipment also needs repairs from time to time, which can be costly and inconvenient.

If the pros outweigh the cons, check out what local sporting stores offer. There are also stores that sell used exercise equipment. Look in the classified ads on Craigslist, eBay, or your local newspaper. You may find a real bargain. Be sure to try out equipment before you buy it. Here's a checklist of questions to ask to get the best products:

- Is the manufacturer reputable? How long has it been in business? What other products does it make?
- Does the equipment come with a warranty? What does it cover? Is there an additional charge for the warranty?

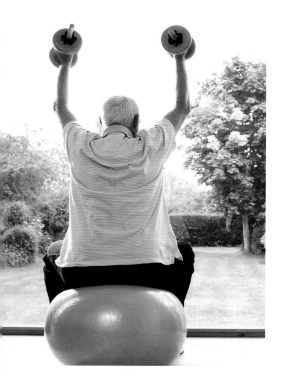

Home exercise equipment makes exercising convenient and carefree.

- Is electricity required to operate the equipment? (Motors and other electronic devices are prone to breaking down.)
- Is the equipment adjustable for all sizes and fitness levels?
- How much does it cost?
- How much space is required to operate it?
- Is it sturdy enough to last for several years?
- Are operating and exercise training instructions provided?
- Can you achieve your physical activity goals with this equipment?
- Is it safe?
- Do you think you would enjoy this equipment for a long time and use it regularly?
-  Go to the ALED Online Web site for more information on choosing the home exercise equipment that is right for you.

Did You Know?

The convenience of having a treadmill at home can make it easier to be active and even lose a few extra pounds. In a study at the University of Pittsburgh (Jakicic, Winters, Lang, and Wing 1999), researchers put 148 overweight women on a diet and assigned them to one of three five-day-a-week exercise programs. The first group walked 40 minutes in a single session. The second and third groups divided their 40 minutes into 10-minute bouts. Women in the third group had an advantage: The researchers gave them treadmills to use at home.

After 18 months, the group exercising at home lost over 16 pounds (7.3 kg). The first and second groups lost nearly 13 pounds (5.9 kg) and 8 pounds (3.6 kg), respectively. Why? Home equipment such as a treadmill may be particularly appealing to people who are overweight and sensitive about how they look at the gym or walking around town. With home exercise equipment, you can work out whenever you want. You can wear whatever you want, too.

This study also showed that regardless of whether you do long or short bouts, the more exercise you get, the more weight you lose. (See the following table.)

If one of your goals is to lose weight or to prevent weight gain, first aim for 150 minutes of moderate activity (or 75 minutes of vigorous activity) weekly. Then start looking for ways to add more activity. And remember, just like the women in this study, you will need to be vigilant in reducing your daily calorie intake from food.

Increased Physical Activity Leads to Greater Weight Loss

Min per week of moderate-intensity exercise	Amount of weight loss in 18 months in lb (kg) if calorie intake remains constant
More than 200	28.8 (13.1)
150-200	18.7 (8.5)
Less than 150	7.7 (3.5)

TV-Based Exercise Programs

The last thing we thought we'd ever do is tell you to turn on the TV. However, some television-based exercise programs are fun and useful, including many available on DVD. Check out the local video store, sporting goods store, or Netflix Web site. If you have cable or satellite service, check out FitTV for a schedule of exercise programs.

The latest advance in TV-based exercise programs is *Wii Fit*, a game that allows users to bowl, play tennis, and even golf in the comfort of their own living rooms. Scientists are just beginning to study how much *Wii Fit* and other active video games increase calorie expenditure. One small study showed that children and adults playing various video games expended more calories playing boxing in the *Wii Sports* game than with the more sedentary, traditional video games (Lanningham-Foster et al. 2009). In another study, adolescents burned more calories playing Wii tennis and Wii bowling in *Wii Sports* than playing sedentary computer games (Graves, Ridgers, and Stratton 2008). Although more research is needed to say that active video games are a winner, they're better than sitting on the couch. And playing a virtual game may get you interested in activities that you can then try in their real versions.

Striving for Increased Benefits

If you've stuck with us this far, you're probably meeting the official public health guidelines for physical activity, which call for accumulating 150 minutes or more of moderate-intensity activity each week (Department of Health and Human Services 2008). That's great, especially if you started out completely sedentary. When people move from being inactive to being even moderately active, they enjoy a big pay-off, as the following chart shows.

But remember, doing a little bit more than the recommended level offers even bigger benefits. Most studies of exercise and health show that the benefits of activ-

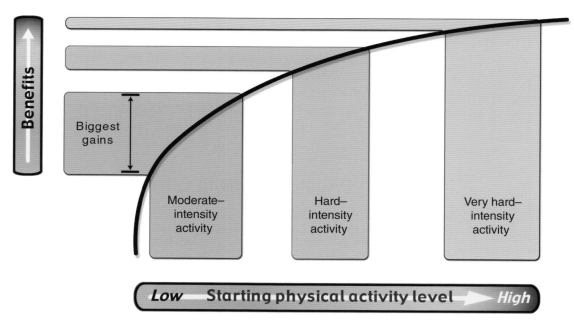

Your greatest health gains will occur when you first start exercising.

Adapted from R.R. Pate, M. Pratt, S.N. Blair, et al. 1995, "Physical activity and public health," *JAMA* 273(5): 402-407.

ity are dose dependent. That's jargon for a simple idea: the more you do, the more benefits you'll get.

Ideally, all of us should do something active every day for at least half an hour. How can you add more activity? You can increase the total time each week you are active, the number of times per day or days per week you are physically active, or the intensity level of your activities. Better yet, you can do all three. Here are examples drawn from the ideas our participants came up with to push a little harder.

Increase Time

- Add an extra 500 steps to your walks.
- Start five minutes ahead of your normal walking time.
- Offer to mow or rake a neighbor's yard.
- After walking, take an extra lap around the block to cool down.
- Before shopping at the mall, take a brisk 15-minute walk.
- Park your car as far away from your destination as possible. You may do away with the stress of finding a close parking space, and you'll add a useful way to expend energy. If you don't drive, get off the bus a stop or two earlier than your destination.
- Instead of having dessert at lunch, take a walk. Invite a friend to come along.

Increase Frequency

- Identify sedentary times that you can convert to active times. Look back to your Personal Time Study to identify opportunities.
- If you walk up and down the stairs at work twice a day, add another roundtrip or two each day.
- In addition to longer stretches of activity, take advantage of two-minute and five-minute opportunities throughout the day.
- While the kids are at soccer practice (or baseball, hockey, marching band, or dance), walk around the field a few times. Don't have kids who play sports? You can still find a field or park to walk around.
- Catch up on active jobs. These include weeding the garden, mowing the lawn (no riding mowers, please), doing home repairs, or doing vigorous housework, such as mopping the floor.

Increase Intensity

- If you feel comfortable doing moderate-intensity activities, start adding more vigorous exercises. Check out appendix C for activities that count as vigorous.
- Celebrate at the end of the day by grooving to whatever music you enjoy. Dance by yourself or with someone you love. If you have a favorite local dance club, go for it. If not, boogie across the living room floor. Make sure you work up a bit of a sweat!
- Pick up the pace of whatever activity you do. Add a little jogging to your walk. Do a series of fast sprints, moderate-pace cycling, fast sprints, and moderate-pace cycling while riding your bike.
- Try a new vigorous sport.

Remember, every minute of vigorous-intensity exercise counts as two minutes of moderate-intensity exercise. You get the same benefits in half the time. Here's another way to think about it. If you do a 30-minute jog instead of a 30-minute walk, you get twice the benefits in the same amount of time.

The Talk Test

Here's a great way to judge whether you are a doing moderate- or vigorous-intensity physical activity. If you can sing a song at the same time you are doing a physical activity, you are at a light intensity. If you can't sing but you can still talk fairly comfortably, you are in the moderate-intensity zone. If you are so breathless that you can't sing or talk, you're doing a high-intensity physical activity.

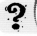 ## Did You Know?

Getting to Work Under Your Own Steam

Not everyone can walk or pedal to work, but those who do may enjoy better health as a result, according to a 2009 study. Scientists at the University of North Carolina at Chapel Hill studied 2,364 adults who worked outside the home. About 17 percent used their own muscle power to get to work, usually walking or bicycling. These active commuters were fitter and enjoyed a healthier weight. They also had better triglyceride, blood pressure, and insulin levels than nonactive commuters (Gordon-Larsen et al. 2009).

Even if you can't pedal or walk all the way to work, you may be able to go part of the way under your own steam. Consider getting off the bus or subway a couple of stops early and walking the rest of the way. If you drive to work, park as far away from your office as you can. Perhaps you can even park on the top deck of a parking garage and then use the stairs. If you don't commute, consider walking or bicycling to the local market instead of driving. Every time you walk or pedal instead of drive, you improve your fitness and health. Using muscle power instead of gas power also offers environmental benefits.

 ## Real Life

For years Paula had wanted a dog. After she retired from teaching, she especially longed for the companionship of a pet. If only she had a dog that needed to be walked, she told herself, she'd be more active. Unfortunately, the apartment she lived in didn't allow dogs.

Then one day, a friend came up with an idea. Since many dog owners were too busy to give their dogs the attention they need, why not set up a dog-walking service? Paula decided to give it a try. She printed up posters and put them around town. It didn't take

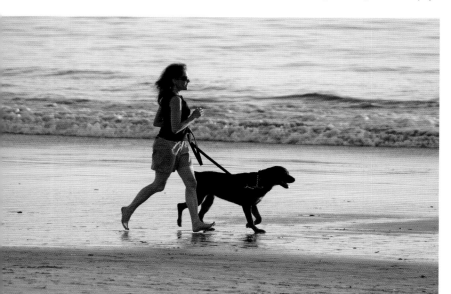

long for the phone to begin ringing, and within several months she had a regular clientele. One owner who worked long hours and often didn't get home until late hired her to walk his collie in the afternoon. Another dog owner, who traveled for work, hired Paula to dog-sit and house-sit whenever she was on the road.

Paula loved every minute of it. Before long she was walking at least an hour a day, often more. Thanks to a clever idea, she was able to combine physical activity with a new part-time job. As if that weren't enough, she finally had a dog—or rather, a dozen dogs—in her life.

Activity Alert

Pushing Harder

All you have to do is feel the number of pages between your thumb and finger to know you're getting close to the end of this book. That's why we've been encouraging you to push just a little harder.

 Many people find it easier to reach a goal if they put it in writing. So get out your pen or pencil—it's commitment time. You can also download a copy of this form from the ALED Online Web site.

My Plan to Push a Little Harder

1. How often do you include at least 150 minutes of physical activity in your weekly schedule? (Circle one.)

   0 times a month   **1-2 times a month**

   3 times a month   **4 or more times a month**

2. Do you plan to increase or maintain your current activity level? (Circle one.)

   Increase   **Maintain**

3. If you are planning to increase your activity level, circle the things you plan to increase:

   Frequency

   Amount of time (duration)

   Intensity

   New types of activities

4. Now list the specific strategies you could use to increase your activity. Remember to be specific.

   _____

   _____

   _____

   _____

5. Pick the strategies you will try this week and put them into the following weekly plan:

Day	Activity and Strategy
Monday	_____
Tuesday	_____
Wednesday	_____
Thursday	_____
Friday	_____
Saturday	_____
Sunday	_____

Weighing In

For years researchers have known that obesity and overweight run in families. A child born to overweight parents is more likely to be overweight than a child born to parents who are not obese. Scientists don't fully understand what inherited characteristics lead people to be more likely to gain weight. Some think the problem may lie in faulty satiety signals, the messages that go from stomach to brain to say, "Enough already, I'm full." Others think that individuals may have different metabolic set points, which determine how much body fat is stored. Genes have been identified that seem to give certain people a heightened preference for sweet foods—so-called sweet-tooth genes. Most likely, a combination of inherited characteristics predisposes certain people to put on too much weight.

Notice the word *predispose*. No one is fated to be fat. Obesity is also determined by the world we live in and the way we live in the world. Most experts think that environment plays a bigger role than heredity. The good news is that you can achieve a healthy weight for your body type, but it means controlling your environment. You can walk instead of drive to the market. You can turn off the TV and do something active instead. You can get together with friends for a pickup game of soccer or volleyball. You can pack a healthy lunch instead of going to a fast-food restaurant. In many ways, you can choose the kind of environment and the kind of life you want to live.

And here is the latest good news on genetics and obesity. Recent research suggests that physical activity may reduce the BMI level (a measure of obesity) that might otherwise be expected due to the presence of a specific obesity gene (Vimaleswaran et al. 2009). So even though you can't change your genes, by being physically active you can turn down some of the obesity genes you might have.

Studies of weight and genes point out a larger truth. All of us are born with certain traits, but we also have the ability to shape our destinies. We may not be able to choose whether we're tall or short, thin or hefty, but we can make choices every day that help ensure good health. One of those choices is to resist the forces that make so many of us sedentary. Once you begin to choose an active lifestyle, the choice becomes a habit that in turn becomes part of who you are. As you feel more comfortable, you can add time, frequency, intensity, and variety to your activities. Many strategies you used earlier to become active can help you push yourself a little harder now.

Need a Boost?

The more active you are, the easier it becomes to think of yourself as an active person. Still, problems can come along that threaten to knock you off track. A busy time at work, a family crisis, an illness, or a period when you feel blah—any of these can get in your way. If you need a little push now and then, here are a few simple ways to motivate yourself:

- Ask someone close to you to help you brainstorm solutions to the issues that are holding you back.
- Keep track of your plans, goals, and activities. Keeping an activity log is a powerful motivator.
- Push yourself to try one or two new activities.
- Explore your home, neighborhood, and work environments to discover new places and ways to be active.
- Each night before you go to bed, write in your calendar when and how you are going to fit in activity the next day.
- Go back to an earlier chapter if you feel the need for a refresher course.

CHAPTER CHECKLIST

Before you move on to the next week's activities, make sure you've done the following:

- Completed the New Opportunities to Be Active form
- Thought about how to get more benefits by pushing a little harder
- Made a plan to increase activity in the weeks to come

 Checked out chapter 10 on the ALED Online Web site for more helpful resources and information for this chapter

References

Bassett, D.R. Jr., P.L. Schneider, and G.E. Huntington. 2004. Physical activity in an Old Order Amish community. *Medicine and Science in Sports and Exercise* 36(1): 79-85.

Department of Health and Human Services. 2008. *Physical activity guidelines for Americans.* Washington, DC: Government Printing Office.

Esparz, J., C. Fox, I.T. Harper, P.H. Bennett, L.O. Schulz, M.E. Valencia, and E. Ravussin. 2000. Daily energy expenditure in Mexican and USA Pima Indians: low physical activity as a possible cause of obesity. *International Journal of Obesity and Related Disorders* 24(1): 55-59.

Gordon-Larsen, P., J. Boone-Heinonen, S. Sidney, B. Sternfeld, D.R. Jacobs, and C.E. Lewis. 2009. Active commuters and cardiovascular disease risk. *Archives of Internal Medicine* 169(13): 1216-1223.

Graves, L.E., N.D. Ridgers, and G. Stratton. 2008. The contribution of upper limb and total body movement to adolescents' energy expenditure whilst playing Nintendo Wii. *European Journal of Applied Physiology* 104(4): 617-623.

Jakicic, J.M., C. Winters, W. Lang, and R.R. Wing. 1999. Effects of intermittent exercise and use of home exercise equipment on adherence, weight loss, and fitness in overweight women: a randomized trial. *Journal of the American Medical Association* 282(16): 1554-1560.

Lanningham-Foster, L., R.C. Foster, S.K. McCrady, T.B. Jensen, N. Mitre, and J.A. Levine. 2009. Activity-promoting video games and increased energy expenditure. *Journal of Pediatrics* 154(6): 819-823.

Vimaleswaran, K.S., S. Ki, H. Zhao, J. Luan, S.A. Bingham, K.T. Khaw, U. Ekelund, N.J. Wareham, and R.J.F. Loos. 2009. Physical activity attenuates the body mass index—increasing influence of genetic variation in the FTO gene. *American Journal of Clinical Nutrition* 90: 425-428.

Chapter
Eleven

Positive Planning

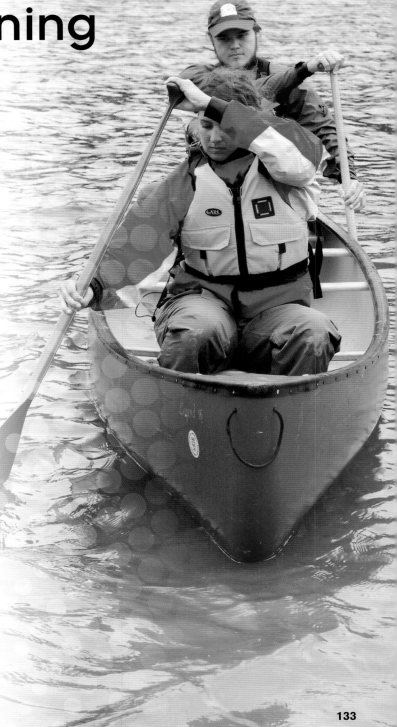

In This Chapter

- Turning negative messages into a positive attitude
- Preparing for situations that can throw you off track
- Planning to increase your activity

By now you've probably begun to think differently about yourself and your life. You've gained confidence that you can plan and follow through on a goal to increase your activity. You may have switched from thinking of yourself as a couch potato to seeing yourself as an active person who enjoys getting up and *doing* something. We certainly hope you've begun to enjoy the benefits, both physically and mentally.

Now's the time to think about how to maintain your active lifestyle for the long haul. In this chapter we'll take another look at strategies to keep your plans flexible, so you can steer clear of trouble and stay on track.

Making It Last

One important advantage of a lifestyle approach to activity is its adaptability. You don't have to worry about finding a gym nearby. You don't have to reserve an hour of your schedule to work out. You don't even have to work up a hard sweat. Lifestyle activity, by its nature, becomes an integral part of your life. For that reason, it's often easier to maintain through life's ups and downs.

As you have learned, many types of physical activity count as exercise. Walking, yard work, climbing stairs, dancing, and playing volleyball with the kids all qualify. As long as physical activity is at least moderate intensity, it will improve your fitness and other measures of good health. You've heard it before: The more you do, the more you'll benefit.

Being active doesn't need to be hard work. It's a natural part of a healthy life. It can even be one of the most pleasurable parts of life.

Your goal after you finish the ALED program is to maintain the physical activity habit you've worked so hard to establish. What will it take? There are many factors, but these top the list:

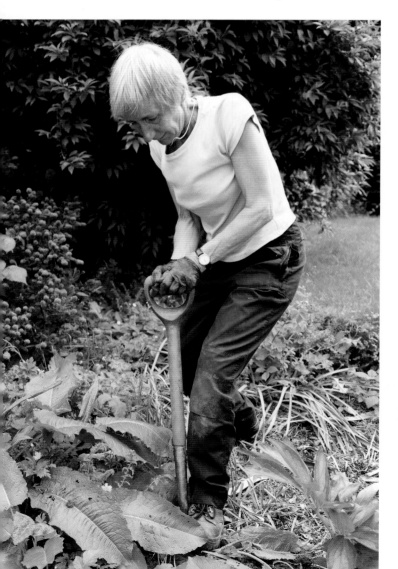

- Making a commitment
- Planning well
- Being flexible
- Staying out of a rut
- Having a positive attitude

Here's why we think these five factors are so important. To change your life for the better, you have to want to change. That's true whether you intend to stop smoking, eat a healthier diet, or become more physically active. Making the commitment to change can help you overcome hurdles and stay on course no matter what obstacles life throws your way. The participants in our program who made lasting changes were those who committed themselves to the goal of becoming more active.

The next step is planning. Whether you want to fit in a five-minute walk or a 5-mile (8 km) hike, the key to making it happen is effective planning. We know from our studies that the people who get in the habit of setting aside time for activity are far more likely to remain active over the long run compared with those who don't plan ahead.

As we've often repeated, the path to making a lifelong change isn't always smooth. If you miss your

Staying fit doesn't have to mean going to the gym or changing your daily schedule.

planned activity for one day, be sure to make a plan for the following day, even if it's a simple five-minute walk. If you are injured, try an alternative activity if you can. If you're sick, wait until you're feeling better and gradually get back to your routine. If there's a problem at home or work, give it the priority it deserves, and resolve to get back to your activities as soon as you can. Set short-term and long-term goals. Find ways around new challenges through problem solving. Remind yourself of all the benefits you've gotten or hope to get from staying active.

It can be good to have a routine, but doing the same thing over and over can get monotonous. Boredom has sidelined many a person's good intentions. That's why we encourage you to add a little excitement by exploring new routes, being active with a variety of people, trying new activities, or increasing the intensity level of your activities.

Finally, we want to emphasize the importance of a positive attitude. Nothing is more discouraging than a voice in your head that says, "I can't." Negative attitudes and all-or-nothing thinking are two of the biggest obstacles many people face. A positive attitude and encouraging mental messages, on the other hand, can go a long way toward helping people get past rocky times. Being positive can help prevent the occasional lapse from turning into a relapse or a total collapse.

 ## Activity Alert

What Do You Think?

If you still find yourself being undermined by negative thoughts that leave you feeling discouraged or even depressed, take a few moments to think about ways to highlight the positive. These four steps should help.

1. Identify the negative thought.

Too many people let negative thoughts take over—as soon as they realize they've lapsed, they collapse and give up. Typical negative thoughts are "I'm a failure," "I'll never be able to stick with my plan," or "I've failed before and I'll probably fail again." Less obvious but equally destructive negative thoughts take the form of "I'm just not cut out for exercise," "It's just not worth all the trouble," "I've always hated exercise," or "It's too hard." If you find yourself slipping back into bad habits, be aware of the thoughts that lead you there.

2. Decide whether the thought is right or wrong. (Hint: It's usually wrong.)

Of course, we want you to take your plan for activity seriously. It's reasonable to be concerned if you've gotten off track for a few weeks in a row. However, you're not a failure because you don't meet your plan one day, one week, or even longer. That's an example of destructive all-or-nothing thinking. We all can be active in a way that suits our temperament and physical abilities, and it's well worth adopting healthy habits.

3. Counter negative thoughts with a more accurate, reasonable, and positive response.

Let's say you find yourself thinking, "I haven't stuck with it, and I'm never going to be able to do it." Instead, tell yourself, "I'm having a setback, but it doesn't have to be permanent. I'm still committed to being active. I know I can do it. I've worked through problems before. I can do it again." Remind yourself of ways you have gotten back on track by reviewing previous weeks in the book. Or let's say you sometimes get discouraged and think, "I'll never be able to do it. I'm destined to fail." In that case, remind yourself that true failure comes only from giving up. As long as you're still trying, you're in the game. Make a list of several things you've succeeded at in your life. Then vow to add one more item to that list: becoming an active person.

4. Make a specific plan.

For instance, decide immediately to put a short walk back into your daily routine. Make a plan to do something active the next weekend. Call on a friend who has helped support your efforts to be more active. Ask for a little more support and encouragement.

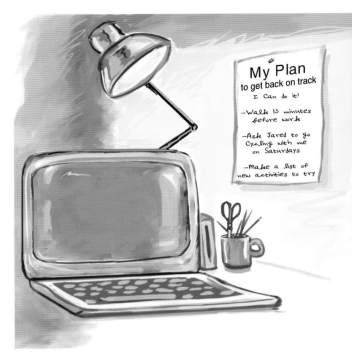

My Plan
to get back on track
I Can do it!

—Walk 15 minutes before work

—Ask Jared to go Cycling with me on Saturdays

—Make a list of new activities to try

 ## Real Life

By the end of our lifestyle program, James had been through so many ups and downs, he felt as if he had been on a roller coaster. At the beginning, he surpassed his expectations, quickly racking up at least 150 minutes of brisk walking each week. Then came a badly sprained knee from a fall when he tripped over his grandson's toy dump truck that knocked him out of commission for three weeks. No sooner was he back to walking 30 minutes a day than a good friend in his retirement community died. Greatly saddened, it was almost a month before his life returned to normal. He was just beginning to get back into an active routine when he caught the flu and lost another week and a half.

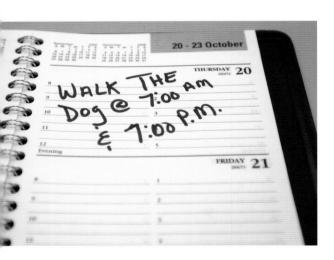

James began to think the whole thing wasn't worth the trouble. He began to say to himself, "This is never going to work." Hearing that voice in his head, he stopped and took stock. First, he told himself that he wasn't a quitter. He knew from experience that if he could get hold of the problem, he could solve it. Using the Great IDEA! form on page 29 in chapter 3, he wrote out the problem and listed ideas for solutions. He began to have insights into his ways of thinking and acting.

Thinking over the past few months, he realized how important planning was. He tended to lose sight of his priorities when he found himself without a plan. He also reminded himself of the benefits of being active. He felt better, his blood pressure and cholesterol levels had fallen, and he had even lost a couple of pounds.

James made a few simple changes. He made a sign that said "No excuses" and put it on the refrigerator at home. He began writing his activity plan on his calendar. After walking, riding a bike, or playing golf with his friends, he took time to notice the pleasant tiredness in his legs and arms. He made a point of enjoying how great it felt to be doing something good for himself.

 ## Did You Know?

It's never too late to reap the benefits of a more active life. That's the good news from a 35-year study by researchers at Uppsala University in Sweden. In the early 1970s, the scientists began to follow a group of 2,205 50-year-old men, checking on their health and lifestyle habits roughly every decade (Byberg et al. 2009). Compared with the least physically active participants, men who consistently engaged in regular moderate-intensity physical activities cut their risk of dying prematurely by 22 percent. The most active men had a 32 percent lower mortality rate.

Here's the especially good news from the study. Ten years after some of the inactive 50-year-olds took up active lifestyles, their risk of dying was the same as men who had been active throughout their lives. Of course, a lifetime of physical activity is ideal. But these results show that even after middle age, adopting a more active lifestyle can undo some of the risks of being sedentary.

 # Activity Alert

Troubleshooting Revisited

 Not quite meeting your goals? There may be an easy way around the problem. Here's an opportunity to do some constructive troubleshooting. You can also download a copy of this form from the ALED Online Web site.

My Plans for Troubleshooting

1. First, think about the barriers in your way. If you aren't managing to follow your plan, why not? List the biggest obstacles.

    a. _____

    b. _____

    c. _____

2. Do you still find yourself discouraged by negative thoughts? (Circle one.)

    Never   Rarely   Sometimes   Always

3. If so, what are they? List the negative messages that get in your way. Then think about ways to counter them and write your positive responses.

    Negative thought   Positive response

    a. _____

    b. _____

    c. _____

4. Do you feel confident that you can maintain your program of physical activity no matter what problems arise? (Circle one.)

    Almost always   Sometimes   Rarely   Almost never

5. If you answered "rarely" or "almost never," think about steps you can take to feel more confident than you do now. One way is to set more realistic short- and long-term goals. Create a specific plan and write it down.

From S.N. Blair, A.L. Dunn, B.H. Marcus, R.A. Carpenter, and P. Jaret, 2011, *Active Living Every Day*, 2nd ed. (Champaign, IL: Human Kinetics).

Weighing In

Setting a goal and working out a plan to reach it is important. Setting an impossible goal, however, can spell trouble. That's especially true when it comes to losing weight. Magazines trumpet miracle diets to help you lose weight fast. Drop 15 pounds (6.8 kg) in one week! Lose inches in a matter of days!

Don't believe it. The healthiest way to lose weight is gradually. Many experts say that if you're overweight, you should set a goal of losing 5 to 10 percent of your current weight. Let's say you weigh 180 pounds (81.6 kg). A reasonable goal would be to lose 9 to 18 pounds (4.1-8.2 kg) at a rate of about 1 pound (.5 kg) a week. Don't be discouraged if you make a little progress and then reach a plateau. That's perfectly normal, according to many weight-loss experts. Most people lose some weight, plateau, and then lose a little more weight, especially if they increase their daily activity level.

If you are getting discouraged, reexamine your goals and ask yourself if they are reasonable. If they are not, set a new goal, one you are pretty confident you can reach. Here's our advice:

- Set a goal to lose just 5 percent of your current weight to start with.
- Plan to lose about .5 to 1 pound (.2-.5 kg) per week.
- Remember that plateaus are normal.
- Keep a positive attitude.
- Increase your physical activity level by increasing the total weekly minutes or steps before you start increasing the intensity. As you become fitter, increase the intensity level.
- Emphasize eating fruits, vegetables, whole grains, and low-fat dairy products. Eat moderate amounts of fat and calories.

 ## Activity Alert

In chapter 3, we asked you to make a list of the hurdles that sometimes stand between you and achieving the goal of being more active. We also asked you to list the benefits you wanted to gain by becoming more physically active. We hope you've found ways around some of those hurdles. We also hope you've begun to reap some of the benefits.

 Now is a good time to review your challenges and the benefits you're getting. Look back to pages 26 and 27. Write out all the challenges you listed back then in the following space. Add any new challenges you have run into since that time. You can also download a copy of this form from the ALED Online Web site.

My Challenges

1. _____
2. _____
3. _____
4. _____
5. _____
6. _____
7. _____
8. _____

Scratch through any of the challenges on your list that are no longer challenges. Many of the participants in our studies came to realize that what they thought were barriers were simply problems they hadn't taken the time to solve. During our program, they developed insights, skills, and strategies that allowed them to remove many of their challenges.

Now write out all the personal benefits you listed in chapter 3 in the following space. You can also download a copy of this form from the ALED Online Web site.

Add any new benefits or positive changes that have occurred since you started the ALED program. Remember, benefits aren't always physical. As you've already seen, one of our participants discovered that he was able to spend more time with his teenage son during evening walks. Another found a new source of income along with a way to be active by setting up a dog-walking service. Take time to consider all the benefits you are getting in your new, more active life.

My Benefits

1. _____
2. _____
3. _____
4. _____
5. _____
6. _____
7. _____
8. _____

From S.N. Blair, A.L. Dunn, B.H. Marcus, R.A. Carpenter, and P. Jaret, 2011, *Active Living Every Day*, 2nd ed. (Champaign, IL: Human Kinetics).

Keeping track of challenges and benefits can help you monitor your progress. It can also give you a renewed sense of confidence that you can overcome problems that get in your way. As a result of your successes, you will feel more confident about being able to work through other challenges in the future.

Keep in mind that some of the benefits of physical activity, such as a feeling of accomplishment, show up quickly. Studies show that some of the overall health benefits of becoming more active can also show up quickly. Blood pressure readings often begin to come down after just a few weeks of physical activity, for example. Improvements in aerobic fitness also begin quickly. Others, such as losing weight, may take longer. The key factor is that you have to stick with being physically active to retain the benefits.

In this chapter, we have explored some of the keys to successful long-term lifestyle change. In the last chapter, we'll help you customize a survival kit that will ensure continuing success in the weeks, months, and years to come.

CHAPTER CHECKLIST

Before you move on to the next week's activities, make sure you've done the following:

- Taken a few moments to identify stubborn negative thoughts and replaced them with positive messages
- Made specific plans for dealing with obstacles that may come along
- Compared your challenges and benefits today with where you started

 Checked out chapter 11 on the ALED Online Web site for more helpful resources and information for this chapter

References

Byberg, L., H. Melhus, J. Sundstrom, A. Ahlbom, B. Zethelius, L.G. Berglund, A. Wolk, and K. Michaelsson. 2009. Total mortality after changes in leisure time physical activity in 50 year old men: 35 years follow-up of population-based cohort. *British Journal of Sports Medicine* 43(7): 482.

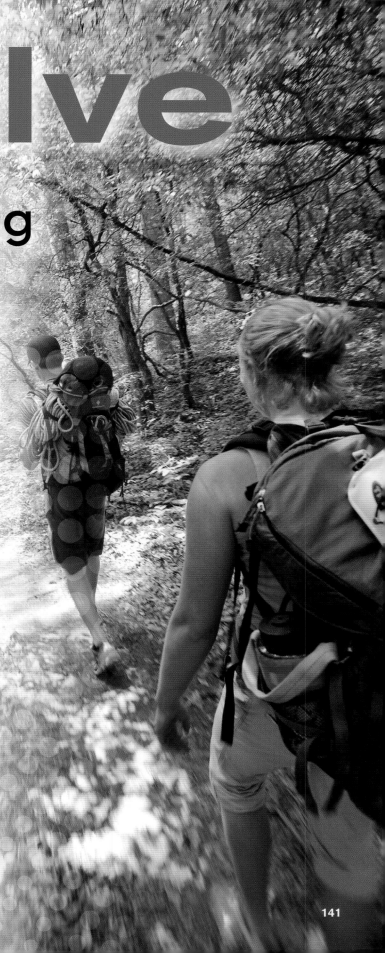

Chapter

Twelve

Making Lasting Changes

In This Chapter

- Celebrating your accomplishments
- Looking back at the activities you like best
- Trying new activities to renew your motivation
- Rating the skills and strategies that work best for you
- Troubleshooting problems that still get in your way
- Making a commitment to the future

The aim of this book is to help you overcome obstacles by using specific skills and to inspire you to become active every day for the rest of your life. Even the best book in the world can only set you on the right path, though. Staying on course depends on you. In this final chapter, you'll have a chance to celebrate how far you've come. You'll also work on ways to make sure your healthy changes last for a lifetime.

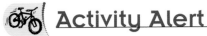

Activity Alert

Positive Changes

Celebrations such as a birthday or the beginning of a new year offer a chance to think about the time gone by and anticipate what lies ahead. You've worked hard at making and keeping a resolution to include activity in your daily life. You deserve to celebrate. Think about what you have accomplished. Review your challenges and benefits in chapter 11, and list your top three benefits here:

Three Reasons to Celebrate

1. _____
2. _____
3. _____

From S.N. Blair, A.L. Dunn, B.H. Marcus, R.A. Carpenter, and P. Jaret, 2011, *Active Living Every Day*, 2nd ed. (Champaign, IL: Human Kinetics).

 You can also download a copy of this form from the ALED Online Web site.

Benefits Keep Growing

More energy, greater self-confidence, lower blood pressure and cholesterol levels, a brighter outlook on life—all are benefits of being physically active. Stay active and those benefits keep adding up. The longer you keep to your goal of getting 150 minutes or more of at least moderate-intensity activity a week, the longer you will retain the benefits. And as you age, these benefits matter even more.

For many people, the experience of making an important and lasting change in their lifestyle gives them insight into themselves. Someone who spends a few hours doing something for a charity, for instance, may be surprised to learn how much she enjoys working with the people of the organization. Someone who tries to quit smoking may be startled to discover how much hard work and motivation it takes to quit for good, and along the way he may uncover unknown reserves of personal strength and commitment. By changing your habits, you change yourself and your view of the world.

We hope you've learned some things about yourself by doing our program. Not all of them have to be positive. There's nothing wrong with discovering that you have to push yourself hard to get up and be active. There is no single strategy or activity that is right for everyone. That's why we encouraged you to brainstorm ways you could become more physically active. We hope what you've learned about yourself has increased your self-confidence.

Activity Alert

What Have You Learned?

Take a moment to think about the past few months. What strengths and weaknesses have you seen in yourself? Write down a few of the most important insights. Getting to know yourself will help you get past the biggest hurdle that lies ahead: making a real and lasting change in your lifestyle. You can also download a copy of the following form from the ALED Online Web site.

Three Things I've Learned About Myself

1. _____
2. _____
3. _____

From S.N. Blair, A.L. Dunn, B.H. Marcus, R.A. Carpenter, and P. Jaret, 2011, *Active Living Every Day*, 2nd ed. (Champaign, IL: Human Kinetics).

 # Real Life

When Hye-Suk joined Project *Active*, he had tried and eventually abandoned so many efforts to shape up and slim down that he'd begun to think of himself as a failure. No sooner would he make a resolution to go on a diet or begin to exercise than a voice in his head would say, "You've never succeeded before. What makes you think you'll do it this time?"

Thinking about obstacles that got in his way, Hye-Suk became aware of the voice in his head. He realized that the discouraging voice was there no matter what he attempted to do. What a revelation that was! Learning to counter those negative messages with positive ones gave Hye-Suk an unexpected sense of possibility. "I can do it if I really want to," he'd tell himself. "Of course people have setbacks," he'd remind himself.

Eventually Hye-Suk reached his goal of being more active. He even grew to enjoy it. And something even more important happened: he banished the negative and demoralizing voice in his head. He came to realize that his negative thoughts weren't true. Worse, they were self-defeating. He learned that he could turn *can't* into *can*. He began to think about himself and his life with confidence and enthusiasm.

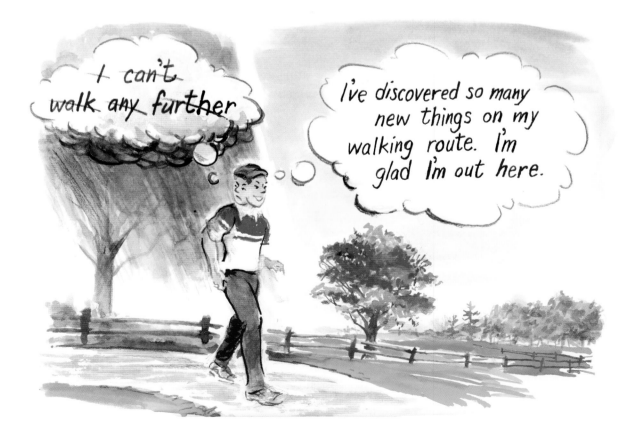

Secrets for Success

Magazines are brimming with stories that offer the secrets to success. Successful weight loss! Ageless beauty! Financial independence! By now you know that there is no one secret to success. Success takes many steps, and people attain their goals in many ways.

Like you, the people in Project *Active* and our other studies tried many strategies for increasing their physical activity. After giving various ideas a fair try, they found that some worked better than others. Here are a few examples:

- Nancy found that her love of nature, specifically walking on trails through the woods near her home, kept her motivated through rain or shine, hot or cold. When she had foot surgery, she had to give up walking for a while. After two months of inactivity, getting started again wasn't easy. She began by walking in the local pool to get back in shape. Fortunately, spring was just beginning. Daffodils were coming up. Trees had begun to leaf out. The attractions of nature were enough to get her back to walking 40 minutes three days per week after work.

- For Charisse, variety was the key to success. Previously when she joined a gym, she quickly tired of the stair machines and treadmills. Now she's learned to love spinning, kickboxing, bicycling, and taking brisk walks through the neighborhood. She and her fiancé have even begun participating in fun runs together.

- Miguel's secret to success can be described in one word: bicycling. He hadn't pedaled a bike since he was in high school. When a friend suggested going on a ride into the country, he decided to give it a try. He had a blast! He scheduled at least three short rides around the neighborhood during the week and one longer ride during the weekends. Now he's training for a 50K ride. "I never would have gotten this far if I hadn't found something I loved to do," he admits.

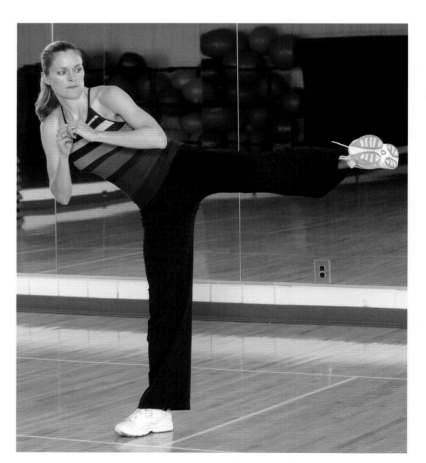

One key to staying active is finding an activity that you enjoy.

Renewing Your Motivation

One way to stay motivated is to get together with other people to share ideas and strategies for adding activities to your daily routine. For example, we asked our Project *Active* participants to bring in items that represented the physical activity they liked to do. We were surprised by what they brought.

One participant brought only a paperback book. That was it. She explained that when she first started to think about being more physically active, she always felt as if she'd rather curl up with a good book. She decided to use her love of reading as her reward for being active. She was able to discipline herself to walk before reading. By the end of the program she was walking 3 miles (4.8 km) a day. She'd also read almost 20 books. Once she felt confident that she could set a goal and meet it, she invested in a stationary bike at home. During cold and wet weather, she could pedal and turn the pages of her book at the same time.

Another participant brought in dozens of items to show-and-tell. Turns out he built his activity around his children. Setting a good example for them was his main motive for becoming more active. The more unusual and zany the activity, the more fun he and his kids had. They roller-skated. They juggled. They even learned to ride a unicycle. Not everyone wants to learn circus tricks to stay active, but playing with your kids or grandchildren can be a rewarding way to add activity to family life.

There are other ways to stay inspired. For starters, look over the list of activities you scouted out in your community in chapter 10. Choose one or two new ones you might like to try. Over the next couple weeks, keep a sharp eye out for what other people are doing to stay active.

Go to the ALED Online Web site to learn about ways you can promote physical activity in your community. Research shows it is easier for people to become and stay active if they live in a setting or among others who support and value an active lifestyle. There is a lot we can do as individuals and in groups to make our worksites, neighborhoods, towns, counties, cities, states, and nation more conducive to moving more for people of all ages. At the ALED Online Web site, you'll find links to resources that will guide you in being a physical activity advocate.

Activity Alert

What's Your Strategy?

Use the form on page 146 to think critically about which skills and strategies worked best for you. Which strategies were important to your success? Which ones weren't important? Give yourself time to think about each one carefully. Put a check mark in the appropriate box for each strategy. You can also download a copy of this form from the ALED Online Web site.

Look over your answers now. Circle the strategies that have made a difference for you. Keep them in mind whenever you hit a rocky stretch. They represent your personal keys to achieving success.

What Works, What Doesn't?

	Very important	Some-what important	Not important
1. Replacing sedentary activities such as watching TV with active ones such as taking short walks			
2. Becoming aware of the benefits of being physically active, especially the ones that most matter to me			
3. Setting short- and long-term goals for becoming and staying active			
4. Rewarding myself for reaching my short- and long-term goals			
5. Getting support from my family and friends			
6. Turning negative thoughts into positive ones			
7. Monitoring how much activity I do every day by counting steps or minutes			
8. Becoming flexible in thinking about what counts as physical activities			
9. Learning new ways to manage my stress and my time better			
10. Finding new opportunities for activity close to my work and home			
11. Planning ahead for situations that might cause me to relapse			

What other strategies have helped you along the way? List them here:

_____

_____

From S.N. Blair, A.L. Dunn, B.H. Marcus, R.A. Carpenter, and P. Jaret, 2011, *Active Living Every Day*, 2nd ed. (Champaign, IL: Human Kinetics).

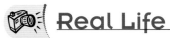 **Real Life**

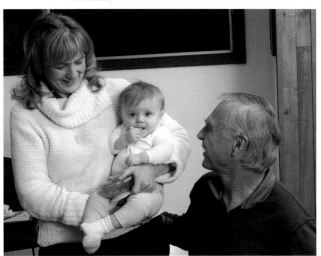

Joyce had watched her mother's health decline and with it her ability to do simple things such as climbing the stairs or loading the dishwasher. Joyce wanted to do everything possible so that she herself would remain active and independent as long as possible. She and her husband were about to retire, and she wanted to make sure she would be able to enjoy it.

At first, it wasn't easy. Joyce had to push herself hard to take even 10-minute walks. The only way she motivated herself was to think of them as a necessity. As she put it, "I'm not thrilled when I brush my teeth, but I wouldn't go a day without doing it! I realize this is something that I'm going to have to work at every day. When my husband and I retire, I want to be able to travel, to play with our grandchildren, and to continue doing all the things I enjoy."

Six months after she finished the program, Joyce contacted us. She was proud to say that she was staying active, even though she'd had a major relapse when her mother became ill and had to be hospitalized. "I started going through the workbook again," she said. "This time I learned some things I hadn't picked up on the first time. It helped to go back and think of what I had learned and why I wanted to be active."

Tips for Troubleshooting

Many participants in our program returned to earlier chapters when they encountered trouble or needed a little encouragement. So keep this book handy, in case you need expert advice or a little nudge in the right direction. Here's a checklist of some common problems that may arise—and where to go for help—as you continue to move forward in the stages of change.

Not enough time in the day to be active?	Look back to chapter 2 and complete a new Personal Time Study form. This will help you identify occasions when you can turn inactivity into activity.
Running into unexpected obstacles?	Look back at chapter 3 and the Great IDEA! form. It will help you identify barriers and formulate a plan to get past them.
Wondering how many calories you're burning?	Use the calorie calculation form in chapter 5 and the chart in appendix C to help you keep track of the number of calories you are burning in various physical activities.
Having trouble setting goals?	Chapter 4 is full of helpful hints for setting reasonable, attainable goals and rewards that will motivate you to move forward.
Looking for support in your efforts to change?	Check out chapter 6, where you'll find useful advice about enlisting the help you need from family and friends and dealing with naggers and saboteurs.
Sidelined by unexpected problems?	The activities in chapter 7 will help you identify and avoid common pitfalls.
Undone by too much stress?	Stress can undermine almost anyone's physical activity efforts. Chapter 9 offers simple ways to defuse even the most stressful situations.
Having trouble managing your time?	Check out the advice in chapter 9 on managing time and setting priorities.
Getting bored with your exercise?	New ideas abound in chapter 10. Also, check out ALED Online for chapter 12 for other ways to make physical activity more than a physical focus in your life.
Feeling down and ready to give up?	Look for strategies and tips for positive thinking in chapters 6 and 11.
Looking for a strategy that works best for you?	Return to your answers to the questionnaire on page 146 of this chapter.

🚲 Activity Alert

Without a book to guide you from week to week, you may find that old sedentary habits creep back. It may begin when you skip a planned walk or drive somewhere instead of bicycling because you're in a hurry. Then you catch a cold, and you decide to wait until you feel better. Before long . . . you get the idea.

If that happens, here's a quick refresher course you can turn to. We've organized it as a seven-day program with something to do each day. Feel free to adapt it to your own needs. Push yourself a little harder if you can. Or give yourself a little more time to complete these activities if you need it. The point is to nudge yourself back into activity. Here's the plan:

Day 1

- Write down the three most important benefits of activity for you.
- Set aside time for a 15-minute walk (or three 5-minute walks).

Day 2

- Write down three reasons why you stopped being as active as you'd like to be.
- Set aside time for a 20-minute walk (or two 10-minute walks).

Day 3

- Look back at your list from yesterday and brainstorm some solutions to the problems you've encountered.
- Practice a few stretching exercises (see pages 73-74 for instructions).
- Take a 20-minute walk (or two 10-minute walks).

Day 4

- Take a 30-minute walk (or two 15-minute walks).
- Repeat the stretching exercises you tried yesterday.
- Write out a plan for putting into practice some of the solutions you came up with yesterday.

Day 5

- Stretch. Use the time to relax and shake off stress.
- Take another 30-minute walk (or two 15-minute walks).
- Add a few strengthening activities (for examples, see pages 88-91).

Day 6

- Stretch.
- Take another 30-minute walk (or two 15-minute walks).
- Write down three ways to add activities to your everyday routine (for examples, see page 127).

Day 7

- Repeat a few of the strengthening activities you did on day 5.
- Take a 30-minute walk (or two 15-minute walks).
- Identify at least three opportunities for being more active (for examples, check out page 122).
- Make a plan for next week and write it down on your calendar. Be specific about what you plan to do and when you'll do it.

From S.N. Blair, A.L. Dunn, B.H. Marcus, R.A. Carpenter, and P. Jaret, 2011, *Active Living Every Day*, 2nd ed. (Champaign, IL: Human Kinetics).

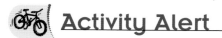 ## Activity Alert

Where Are You Now?

With our program almost at an end, it's a good time to check your readiness to change. By now, you're a pro at completing the questionnaire. Give it another go.

Assessing My Stage of Change

Goal: To do physical activity or exercise regularly, such as accumulating

- 150 min of moderate physical activity per week, or
- 75 min of vigorous physical activity per week, or
- a combination of moderate and vigorous physical activity each week, such as
  - a. 75 min of moderate and 40 min of vigorous physical activity, or
  - b. 90 min of moderate and 25 min of vigorous physical activity.

Moderate-Intensity Activity Examples

- Brisk walking
- Biking <10 mph (16 kph)
- Ballroom dancing
- General gardening, such as weeding
- Golfing (no cart)
- Any other physical activity where the exertion is similar to these

Vigorous-Intensity Activity Examples

- Jogging, running
- Tennis
- Biking >10 mph (16 kph)
- Aerobic dancing
- Heavy gardening, such as digging
- Any other physical activity where the exertion is similar to these

Regular physical activity means meeting or exceeding the physical activity goal described above.

For each statement, please mark *yes* or *no*.

1. I am currently physically active (at least 30 minutes per week). ❑ Yes ❑ No
2. I intend to become more physically active in the next 6 months. ❑ Yes ❑ No
3. I currently engage in **regular** physical activity. ❑ Yes ❑ No
4. I have been **regularly** physically active for the past 6 months. ❑ Yes ❑ No

Scoring Key

- *No* to 1, 2, 3, and 4 = **Precontemplation** stage
- *No* to 1, 3, and 4, *Yes* to 2 = **Contemplation** stage
- *Yes* to 1 and 2, *No* to 3 and 4 = **Preparation** stage
- *Yes* to 1 and 3, *Yes* or *No* to 2, *No* to 4 = **Action** stage
- *Yes* to 1, 3, and 4, *Yes* or *No* to 2 = **Maintenance** stage

From S.N. Blair, A.L. Dunn, B.H. Marcus, R.A. Carpenter, and P. Jaret, 2011, *Active Living Every Day*, 2nd ed. (Champaign, IL: Human Kinetics). Adapted from B.H. Marcus and L.R. Simkin, 1993, "The stages of exercise behavior," *Journal of Sports Medicine and Physical Fitness* 33: 83-88. By permission of B.H. Marcus.

Have you progressed to a new stage since chapter 7? Is your stage different from chapter 1? If you have moved forward, good for you! Remind yourself of the skills you have used to make lasting changes. If you are at the same stage as you were before, take heart. Some stages take several weeks or months to work through. It's even common for some people to backtrack now and then. As long as you remain committed to an active life, you're making progress.

After you complete this book, you may want to revisit the Assessing My Stage of Change questionnaire from time to time to see how you are doing.

What We've Learned

Our research and that of many other scientists around the world has demonstrated the remarkable benefits of an active lifestyle. Research has also offered important insights into how people change their behavior. That work provides useful strategies to help people give up bad habits and adopt healthy ones. Here's a quick checklist of the important insights we've shared with you in this book. Think about each one and how it applies to your experiences since you began:

- Doing at least 150 minutes of moderate-intensity activity each week can lower disease risk and help keep most people fit. That's as simple as 30 minutes of brisk walking on five days per week.

- Doing at least 75 minutes of vigorous-intensity activity each week can also lower disease risk and increase fitness. For people who are sedentary, doing moderate-intensity activity is a good place to start. Gradually adding more minutes of activity and including more vigorous activities will increase the health and fitness benefits.

- Exercise doesn't have to be continuous. Start with 2-minute or 5-minute bouts, and build up to activity bouts of at least 10 minutes. Three 10-minute walks are just as good as one 30-minute walk.

- Readiness to change varies from person to person. Don't worry about comparing your progress through the stages of readiness with someone else's.

- The process of change takes place in stages. The process takes longer for some people than for others.

- Developing skills such as setting short-term and long-term goals and thinking positively can help people maintain an active lifestyle over the long term.

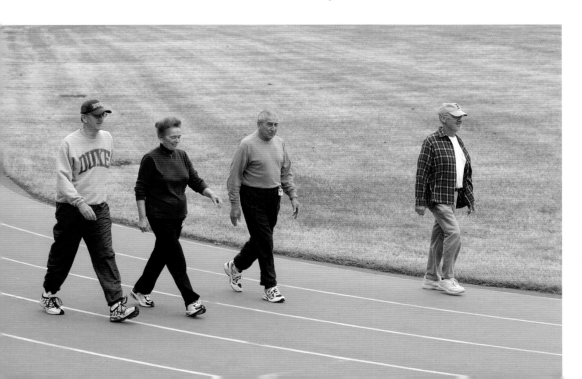

Some people stay motivated by finding friends who enjoy being active.

- Planning how to meet your goal is essential to successful lifestyle change.

- Everyone experiences setbacks on the path to change. People who succeed in the long term learn to view setbacks as learning experiences. One key to success is anticipating problems and having solutions prepared before they happen.

- Being physically active at moderate to high levels is a crucial part of losing weight and keeping it off. Eating a healthy diet is vital as well.

- The more active you are, the bigger the payoff in health, fitness, and outlook. After you become consistent with 150 minutes per week of moderate-intensity activity or 75 minutes per week of vigorous-intensity activity, consider pushing yourself to a higher level. Getting 300 minutes of moderate activity or 150 minutes of vigorous activity per week provides even more health, weight-management, and functional benefits.

 ## Did You Know?

High blood pressure is the leading cause of preventable death among American women. Being active every day can help dramatically decrease the danger. In 2009, researchers from the Harvard School of Public Health reported on a study of 12,319 women who were followed for 14 years (Forman, Stampfer, and Curhan 2009). The scientists found that staying at a healthy weight, doing vigorous physical activities regularly, eating a healthy diet, and following other basic health advice lowered the risk of high blood pressure by 80 percent. Women who were obese or overweight had almost five times the risk of developing high blood pressure, but being physically active significantly reduced the risk.

Parting Words

The focus of this book has been helping you to develop the tools and know-how to become physically active. There is much more you can learn about exercise and physical activity, and there are many other ways in which you can make physical activity a part of your life. For example, you may want to share what you have learned in your physical activity journey with others. If so, you could become an ALED facilitator. Or you may want to share information with your neighborhood association. Perhaps you might even want to write to your local city council to request better parks and paths in your community. Go to the ALED Online Web site for this chapter for a great resource to travel a little farther down the path of making physical activity last a lifetime.

In the end, the one thing you need to maintain an active lifestyle is commitment. So we'd like to ask you to do one more thing before you close the book. Think for a few moments about where you'd like to be three months from now. What kinds of activities would you like to be doing? How often? What barriers would you like to overcome?

When you have your answer, take a piece of paper and write it down in the form of a commitment you make with yourself. It could be as simple as, "Walk at least 45 minutes a day, five days a week," or "Stick to my goals through the coming holidays." It could be a resolution such as, "Don't let negative thoughts get in my way, even when I'm stressed out." Or perhaps it could be something practical, such as "Join an indoor water aerobics class during the winter months," or "Encourage a few of my coworkers to become active this year." If you're feeling confident, write down two or three promises to yourself.

Now take the paper and tape it somewhere prominent, such as on your computer screen at work or the refrigerator door at home. This is your pledge to yourself. With your newfound confidence and skills, you can make it happen.

If this book has taught you one thing, we hope it's this: the effort it takes to become active is richly rewarded by the many benefits. Keep up the good work!

References

Forman, J.P., M.J. Stampfer, and G.C. Curhan. 2009. Diet and lifestyle risk factors associated with incident hypertension in women. *Journal of the American Medical Association* 302(4): 437-439.

Appendix A
Signs and Symptoms of Heart Attack and Stroke

If you or a loved one experiences any of these symptoms, call 911 or your local emergency number immediately. Treatment is often more effective if given quickly.

Heart Attack Warning Signs

- Pressure, fullness, squeezing, or crushing pain in the middle of the chest that lasts more than a few minutes or that goes away and comes back
- Pain that spreads to the shoulders, arms, back, neck, or jaw
- Lightheadedness, dizziness, or fainting
- Unexplained, profuse or intense sweating
- Unusual stomach or abdominal pain
- Nausea or vomiting
- Shortness of breath and difficulty breathing
- Unexplained anxiety, sense of impending doom, weakness, or fatigue
- Palpitations, cold sweat, or paleness

Not every heart attack produces chest pain. Women usually experience the same pain, pressure, and other symptoms as men do, but the tendency of women and their doctors is to ascribe it to something other than a heart attack. All people should take these symptoms seriously.

Stroke Warning Signs

- Sudden but often temporary numbness or weakness of the face, arm, or leg, especially on one side of the body
- Sudden language problems, such as slurred or difficult speech or seeming to be confused
- Sudden visual disturbances, such as blocked or partial loss of vision in one or both eyes
- Abrupt and profound trouble walking, dizziness, or loss of balance or coordination
- Sudden massive headache with no known cause

Appendix B
Stages on the Way to Becoming Active

Change doesn't happen overnight. Most people go through five stages on the way to making any kind of lasting change, whether it's becoming active, kicking the smoking habit, or adopting a new diet. These are the five stages of change involved in becoming active:

1. Not even thinking about being active (precontemplation)
2. Giving it a thought now and then, but not doing it (contemplation)
3. Doing it irregularly (preparation)
4. Doing the new habit consistently but for less than six months (action)
5. Maintaining the new habit for six months or more (maintenance)

Take a careful look at the five stages and identify where you are now. Be honest. In the following five sections, we'll help you identify strategies for moving ahead to the next stage and closer to the goal of becoming active. In our studies at Brown University, these strategies have helped people like you to become more active.

Stage 1: Do I Need This?

Not Even Thinking About Being Active

If you are at stage 1, you haven't become convinced that being active is worth the effort. You don't have any plans to get up and get moving.

If you're like most people at stage 1, the list of reasons you have *not* to exercise is longer than the list of reasons why you want to increase your activity. Some reasons include the following:

- "I don't have time to increase my activity."
- "I don't like to exercise."
- "I tried in the past, and I didn't get anything but sore muscles."
- "I'm too tired to exercise."

We'd like to convince you that you can overcome these reasons. We'd also like to persuade you that there are more good reasons to become active than to stay inactive. These include the following:

- Activity can be fun.
- It's good for you.
- Physical activity can improve your blood cholesterol level.
- Moderate-intensity activity can reduce or even prevent high blood pressure.

Material from copyrighted manual (Do I Need This?; Try It, You'll Like It; I'm on My Way; Keep It Going; and I Won't Stop Now), developed by Bess H. Marcus, PhD, and colleagues of the Miriam Hospital, RI, has been adapted with permission. For more information, contact LSExercise@lifespan.org or call 401-793-3729.

- Physical activity helps in preventing and treating diabetes.
- Adding everyday activity can help you maintain a healthy weight.
- Physical activity is a great stress reliever.
- Regular exercise can decrease feelings of sadness and depression.

 ## Activity Alert

Think about the barriers and benefits of physical activity by using the following questions. Start with the barriers. What do you think?

1	2	3	4	5				
Disagree strongly	Disagree somewhat	Neutral	Agree somewhat	Agree strongly				

	1	2	3	4	5
1. Regular exercise would take too much of my time.					
2. At the end of the day, I am much too tired to exercise.					
3. I would have less time for my family and friends if I exercised regularly.					
Add your answers to the last 3 questions. Total: [＿＿＿＿＿＿]					
This is your *barriers* score.					

Now think about some positive statements about physical activity.

	1	2	3	4	5
1. I would feel better about myself if I became active.					
2. I would feel less stressed if I exercised regularly.					
3. I would feel more comfortable with my body if I became active.					
Add your answers to the last 3 questions. Total: [＿＿＿＿＿＿]					
This is your *benefits* score.					

From S.N. Blair, A.L. Dunn, B.H. Marcus, R.A. Carpenter, and P. Jaret, 2011, *Active Living Every Day*, 2nd ed. (Champaign, IL: Human Kinetics). Material from copyrighted manual (Do I Need This?; Try It, You'll Like It; I'm on My Way; Keep It Going; and I Won't Stop Now), developed by Bess H. Marcus, PhD, and colleagues of the Miriam Hospital, RI, has been adapted with permission. For more information, contact LSExercise@lifespan.org or call 401-793-3729.

Which score is higher—the barriers or the benefits?

If you scored higher on benefits, that means you're becoming convinced that being active is important enough to make the effort. To move forward, talk to friends or family members who make activity a regular part of their lives. Ask them what they do and what benefits they gain. Ask for their advice about simple ways to get started.

If your barriers score was higher, take time this week to list all the good things you can think of about an active lifestyle. What benefits of activity would be most important to you? Also think about the reasons you have for not being more active than you are now. Begin to think about ways you might work around them.

Stage 2: Try It, You'll Like It

Giving Physical Activity a Thought Now and Then, but Not Doing It

If you're at stage 2 on the path to an active life, you're already thinking seriously about becoming active. That's great. Now is the time to consider ways to turn that good intention into action.

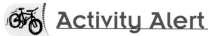 ## Activity Alert

Use the four Ws to begin planning for activity. Circle your answer for each question, or add an answer of your own.

What activity would you be willing to try?
(Think about things you've enjoyed doing in the past or activities that look like fun.)

| Walking | Gardening | Bicycling | Swimming | Dancing | Other |

When could you find 10 minutes to be active?

| In the morning | At lunch | After work | After dinner | Other |

Where is the best place for you to be active?

| At home | In the neighborhood | At the health club | Other |

Whom do you want to be active with?

Just myself | Friends from work
My spouse or partner | My family | Other

From S.N. Blair, A.L. Dunn, B.H. Marcus, R.A. Carpenter, and P. Jaret, 2011, *Active Living Every Day*, 2nd ed. (Champaign, IL: Human Kinetics). Material from copyrighted manual (Do I Need This?; Try It, You'll Like It; I'm on My Way; Keep It Going; and I Won't Stop Now), developed by Bess H. Marcus, PhD, and colleagues of the Miriam Hospital, RI, has been adapted with permission. For more information, contact LSExercise@lifespan.org or call 401-793-3729.

Use your answers to begin to create a plan. If you want to try walking and morning is the best time for you, schedule a time this week to try it. Encourage your significant other or a friend to join you if you prefer to have company, or strike out on your own if you'd rather go solo. Enjoy yourself!

Stage 3: On My Way

Doing Physical Activity Irregularly

If you're at stage 3, you are active now and then, but you haven't been able to make a regular habit of it. Don't be discouraged. You're already well on the way. Now is the time to think about ways to encourage yourself to become regularly active.

 ## Activity Alert

Start by thinking about times recently when you became inactive for too long. What happened? What obstacles got in your way? List a few of the most difficult hurdles you faced.

Obstacle 1 _____

Obstacle 2 _____

Obstacle 3 _____

From S.N. Blair, A.L. Dunn, B.H. Marcus, R.A. Carpenter, and P. Jaret, 2011, *Active Living Every Day*, 2nd ed. (Champaign, IL: Human Kinetics). Material from copyrighted manual (Do I Need This?; Try It, You'll Like It; I'm on My Way; Keep It Going; and I Won't Stop Now), developed by Bess H. Marcus, PhD, and colleagues of the Miriam Hospital, RI, has been adapted with permission. For more information, contact LSExercise@lifespan.org or call 401-793-3729.

Now brainstorm solutions to these obstacles. Here are some suggestions:

- If you find it hard to remember to exercise, put a note on your calendar at work to remind yourself. Leave your walking shoes by the door at home as a reminder.
- If you become inactive when the weather is bad, develop a backup plan. You can walk at the mall on rainy days, for instance. If you live where the winters are long and cold, look into buying home exercise equipment.
- If you stopped exercising because you weren't in the mood, remember that activity improves people's moods. It not only relieves stress but also helps fight sadness and depression. Push yourself to get up and get moving even if you're in a bad mood. Doing a little is better than doing nothing.

Look back at your list of obstacles, and write down at least one possible solution. The next time you find yourself falling off the activity wagon, use these ideas to help get back on track.

Remember to reward yourself often for a job well done. Set a goal of being active almost every day for the next two weeks. If you do so, celebrate by treating yourself to something special.

Stage 4: Sticking to It

Doing the New Habit Consistently but for Less Than Six Months

If you're at stage 4, you are active almost every day, but you haven't managed yet to get beyond the six-month mark. No problem. There are simple strategies that will help you turn activity into a lifelong habit.

- **Set goals.** This is one of the best ways to stay focused and motivated. Think about what you want to accomplish over the next month and then decide what you need to do to get there. Make your goal simple and reasonable enough that you can reach it. Then break the work down into small, easy tasks. Each task is a short-term goal. As you perform each short-term goal, you will move another step toward your long-term goal. Remember to reward yourself when you accomplish your goals.

- **Try a variety of activities.** One obstacle many people face is boredom. After a time, the thrill of walking through the same neighborhood streets begins to wear off. Swimming is wonderful exercise, but every once in a while it's fun to try something else. If you'd rather not change your activities, at least change the setting. Discover a new neighborhood to walk or bicycle in. Try a different swimming stroke, or join a water aerobics class. Another way to prevent your activity routine from becoming boring is to exercise with a friend.

- **Think about your past successes.** By this time, you've had plenty of weeks when you've been active almost every day. You've also had some weeks when it has been hard for you to overcome the obstacles to exercising. What methods did you use to get past those hurdles? How did it feel to reach your short-term goals? Remind yourself that you can make it if you try.

- **Choose a role model.** One way to motivate yourself is to find someone you look up to—someone at work or in your family who has made exercise a lifelong habit. Sit down and tell this person about your goal to increase your activity. Ask for advice. If you don't have someone to talk to, consider joining a club that offers your favorite activity. You may make a few friends who will motivate you. Along the way, you'll be able to give them a little extra push as well.

Stage 5: I'm on Track

Maintaining the New Habit for Six Months or More

If you're at stage 5, you have been active almost every day for six months or more. Congratulations—you're well on your way to making activity a lifelong habit.

This book is full of advice to help you overcome any obstacles you may encounter. Keep it handy just in case you need help along the way. With a long record of success behind you, you can feel confident that you can make it if you stay focused on your goal of staying active.

If you find yourself becoming inactive for a week or two, it's important to understand why and push yourself to get up and get moving. Otherwise you could lose the exercise habit. If this happens to you, make a plan to become active as soon as possible. Set a date and choose a specific activity. Once you've taken one walk or participated in one aerobics class, the next ones will be easier.

Now that you've proven you can do it, take time to encourage a friend or family member to become active. Be a mentor, and you'll find new reasons to stay active yourself.

Activity Alert

To be ready for any obstacles that may come along, take a few minutes to answer some questions.

1. Have you ever stopped being active for a week or more in the past?

2. What caused you to stop?

3. What did you do to get started again?

4. What obstacles are likely to be a problem for you now?

5. What can you do to prepare for those obstacles?

6. What will help you get back on track if you stop being active?

If you run into trouble in the future, look back at your answers. They could encourage you to get moving again. Meanwhile, keep up the good work, and enjoy the many benefits of an active life!

Appendix C
Energy Expenditure Chart

		Estimated calories burned per minute of activity based on an individual's body weight								
	kg	55	64	73	82	91	100	109	118	127
Activities	**lb**	120	140	160	180	200	220	240	260	280
Light										
Child care, sitting or kneeling		2.4	2.8	3.2	3.6	4.0	4.4	4.8	5.2	5.6
Cleaning sink, tub, or toilet		2.4	2.8	3.2	3.6	4.0	4.4	4.8	5.2	5.6
Cleaning, light (dusting, picking up)		2.4	2.8	3.2	3.6	4.0	4.4	4.8	5.2	5.6
Cooking		1.9	2.2	2.6	2.9	3.2	3.5	3.8	4.1	4.4
Fishing, boat		2.4	2.8	3.2	3.6	4.0	4.4	4.8	5.2	5.6
Fishing, ice		1.9	2.2	2.6	2.9	3.2	3.5	3.8	4.1	4.4
Hand sewing		1.9	2.2	2.6	2.9	3.2	3.5	3.8	4.1	4.4
Horseback riding at a walk		2.4	2.8	3.2	3.6	4.0	4.4	4.8	5.2	5.6
Ironing		2.2	2.6	2.9	3.3	3.7	4.0	4.4	4.7	5.1
Mowing lawn, riding mower		2.4	2.8	3.2	3.6	4.0	4.4	4.8	5.2	5.6
Pistol or trap shooting		2.4	2.8	3.2	3.6	4.0	4.4	4.8	5.2	5.6
Playing catch		2.4	2.8	3.2	3.6	4.0	4.4	4.8	5.2	5.6
Playing croquet		2.4	2.8	3.2	3.6	4.0	4.4	4.8	5.2	5.6
Playing pool		2.4	2.8	3.2	3.6	4.0	4.4	4.8	5.2	5.6
Shopping		2.2	2.6	2.9	3.3	3.7	4.0	4.4	4.7	5.1
Sitting, playing cards, at sporting event, in meetings		1.4	1.7	1.9	2.2	2.4	2.6	2.9	3.1	3.3
Sitting, typing or writing		1.7	2.0	2.3	2.6	2.9	3.2	3.4	3.7	4.0
Sleeping		0.9	1.0	1.1	1.3	1.4	1.6	1.7	1.9	2.0
Standing		1.7	2.0	2.3	2.6	2.9	3.2	3.4	3.7	4.0
Stretching		2.4	2.8	3.2	3.6	4.0	4.4	4.8	5.2	5.6
Walking, 30 min per mi (1.6 km)		2.4	2.8	3.2	3.6	4.0	4.4	4.8	5.2	5.6
Washing dishes, standing		2.2	2.6	2.9	3.3	3.7	4.0	4.4	4.7	5.1
Watching TV, sitting or lying		1.0	1.1	1.3	1.4	1.6	1.8	1.9	2.1	2.2

(continued)

(continued)

		kg	55	64	73	82	91	100	109	118	127
					Estimated calories burned per minute of activity based on an individual's body weight							
Activities		**lb**	**120**	**140**	**160**	**180**	**200**	**220**	**240**	**260**	**280**
Moderate											
Aerobic dance, low impact			4.8	5.6	6.4	7.2	8.0	8.8	9.5	10.3	11.1
Archery			3.4	3.9	4.5	5.0	5.6	6.1	6.7	7.2	7.8
Badminton			4.3	5.0	5.7	6.5	7.2	7.9	8.6	9.3	10.0
Bicycling, 10 mph (16 kph)			3.9	4.5	5.1	5.7	6.4	7.0	7.6	8.3	8.9
Bowling			2.9	3.4	3.8	4.3	4.8	5.3	5.7	6.2	6.7
Canoeing			3.9	4.5	5.1	5.7	6.4	7.0	7.6	8.3	8.9
Carpentry, general			2.9	3.4	3.8	4.3	4.8	5.3	5.7	6.2	6.7
Carrying small children			2.9	3.4	3.8	4.3	4.8	5.3	5.7	6.2	6.7
Dancing, line, polka, or country			4.3	5.0	5.7	6.5	7.2	7.9	8.6	9.3	10.0
Dancing, waltz, foxtrot, or samba			2.9	3.4	3.8	4.3	4.8	5.3	5.7	6.2	6.7
Fishing, from bank			3.4	3.9	4.5	5.0	5.6	6.1	6.7	7.2	7.8
Kayaking			4.8	5.6	6.4	7.2	8.0	8.8	9.5	10.3	11.1
Laying sod			4.8	5.6	6.4	7.2	8.0	8.8	9.5	10.3	11.1
Mopping, vacuuming			3.4	3.9	4.5	5.0	5.6	6.1	6.7	7.2	7.8
Mowing lawn, power mower			4.3	5.0	5.7	6.5	7.2	7.9	8.6	9.3	10.0
Painting, exterior			4.8	5.6	6.4	7.2	8.0	8.8	9.5	10.3	11.1
Painting, interior			2.9	3.4	3.8	4.3	4.8	5.3	5.7	6.2	6.7
Playing Frisbee, light			2.9	3.4	3.8	4.3	4.8	5.3	5.7	6.2	6.7
Playing golf, no cart			4.3	5.0	5.7	6.5	7.2	7.9	8.6	9.3	10.0
Playing in marching band			3.9	4.5	5.1	5.7	6.4	7.0	7.6	8.3	8.9
Playing shuffleboard			2.9	3.4	3.8	4.3	4.8	5.3	5.7	6.2	6.7
Playing softball			4.8	5.6	6.4	7.2	8.0	8.8	9.5	10.3	11.1
Raking lawn			3.9	4.5	5.1	5.7	6.4	7.0	7.6	8.3	8.9
Skateboarding			4.8	5.6	6.4	7.2	8.0	8.8	9.5	10.3	11.1
Snorkeling			4.8	5.6	6.4	7.2	8.0	8.8	9.5	10.3	11.1
Snowmobiling			3.4	3.9	4.5	5.0	5.6	6.1	6.7	7.2	7.8
Sweeping sidewalk			3.9	4.5	5.1	5.7	6.4	7.0	7.6	8.3	8.9
Swimming, treading water			3.9	4.5	5.1	5.7	6.4	7.0	7.6	8.3	8.9
Table tennis			3.9	4.5	5.1	5.7	6.4	7.0	7.6	8.3	8.9
Tai chi			3.9	4.5	5.1	5.7	6.4	7.0	7.6	8.3	8.9
Trampoline			3.4	3.9	4.5	5.0	5.6	6.1	6.7	7.2	7.8
Trimming shrubs, manual clipper			4.3	5.0	5.7	6.5	7.2	7.9	8.6	9.3	10.0
Walking, 15 min per mi (1.6 km)			4.8	5.6	6.4	7.2	8.0	8.8	9.5	10.3	11.1
Walking, 20 min per mi (1.6 km)			3.2	3.7	4.2	4.7	5.3	5.8	6.3	6.8	7.3
Washing and waxing automobile			2.9	3.4	3.8	4.3	4.8	5.3	5.7	6.2	6.7
Water aerobics			3.9	4.5	5.1	5.7	6.4	7.0	7.6	8.3	8.9
Weeding, digging in garden			4.3	5.0	5.7	6.5	7.2	7.9	8.6	9.3	10.0

		55	64	73	82	91	100	109	118	127
	kg	55	64	73	82	91	100	109	118	127

Estimated calories burned per minute of activity based on an individual's body weight

Activities	lb	120	140	160	180	200	220	240	260	280
Vigorous										
Aerobic dance, high impact		6.7	7.8	8.9	10.0	11.1	12.3	13.4	14.5	15.6
Bicycling, 12-14 mph (19-23 kph)		7.7	9.0	10.2	11.5	12.7	14.0	15.3	16.5	17.8
Bicycling, 16-19 mph (26-31 kph)		11.6	13.4	15.3	17.2	19.1	21.0	22.9	24.8	26.7
Canoeing, vigorous effort		11.6	13.4	15.3	17.2	19.1	21.0	22.9	24.8	26.7
Carpentry (fence building, roofing)		5.8	6.7	7.7	8.6	9.6	10.5	11.4	12.4	13.3
Chopping wood		5.8	6.7	7.7	8.6	9.6	10.5	11.4	12.4	13.3
Circuit training		7.7	9.0	10.2	11.5	12.7	14.0	15.3	16.5	17.8
Cross-country skiing		8.7	10.1	11.5	12.9	14.3	15.8	17.2	18.6	20.0
Digging ditches		8.2	9.5	10.9	12.2	13.5	14.9	16.2	17.6	18.9
Fishing, wading in stream		5.8	6.7	7.7	8.6	9.6	10.5	11.4	12.4	13.3
Horseback riding at trot		6.3	7.3	8.3	9.3	10.4	11.4	12.4	13.4	14.4
Horseback riding, galloping		7.7	9.0	10.2	11.5	12.7	14.0	15.3	16.5	17.8
In-line skating		12.0	14.0	16.0	17.9	19.9	21.9	23.8	25.8	27.8
Judo, karate, kickboxing		9.6	11.2	12.8	14.4	15.9	17.5	19.1	20.7	22.2
Marching, speedwalking		6.3	7.3	8.3	9.3	10.4	11.4	12.4	13.4	14.4
Mountain biking		8.2	9.5	10.9	12.2	13.5	14.9	16.2	17.6	18.9
Moving furniture		5.8	6.7	7.7	8.6	9.6	10.5	11.4	12.4	13.3
Mowing lawn, hand mower		5.8	6.7	7.7	8.6	9.6	10.5	11.4	12.4	13.3
Playing American football		7.7	9.0	10.2	11.5	12.7	14.0	15.3	16.5	17.8
Playing basketball		7.7	9.0	10.2	11.5	12.7	14.0	15.3	16.5	17.8
Playing handball		11.6	13.4	15.3	17.2	19.1	21.0	22.9	24.8	26.7
Playing hockey, field or ice		7.7	9.0	10.2	11.5	12.7	14.0	15.3	16.5	17.8
Playing racquetball, casual		6.7	7.8	8.9	10.0	11.1	12.3	13.4	14.5	15.6
Playing racquetball, competitive		9.6	11.2	12.8	14.4	15.9	17.5	19.1	20.7	22.2
Playing tennis, doubles		5.8	6.7	7.7	8.6	9.6	10.5	11.4	12.4	13.3
Playing tennis, singles		7.7	9.0	10.2	11.5	12.7	14.0	15.3	16.5	17.8
Playing soccer		9.6	11.2	12.8	14.4	15.9	17.5	19.1	20.7	22.2
Playing volleyball		7.7	9.0	10.2	11.5	12.7	14.0	15.3	16.5	17.8
Rowing, moderate effort		6.7	7.8	8.9	10.0	11.1	12.3	13.4	14.5	15.6
Rowing, vigorous effort		11.6	13.4	15.3	17.2	19.1	21.0	22.9	24.8	26.7
Running, 8 min per mi (1.6 km)		12.0	14.0	16.0	17.9	19.9	21.9	23.8	25.8	27.8
Running, 10 min per mi (1.6 km)		9.6	11.2	12.8	14.4	15.9	17.5	19.1	20.7	22.2
Sawing wood by hand		6.7	7.8	8.9	10.0	11.1	12.3	13.4	14.5	15.6
Shoveling, light to moderate		6.3	7.3	8.3	9.3	10.4	11.4	12.4	13.4	14.4
Skating, roller or ice		6.7	7.8	8.9	10.0	11.1	12.3	13.4	14.5	15.6
Ski machine		6.7	7.8	8.9	10.0	11.1	12.3	13.4	14.5	15.6
Skiing, downhill, moderate effort		5.8	6.7	7.7	8.6	9.6	10.5	11.4	12.4	13.3

(continued)

(continued)

		kg	55	64	73	82	91	100	109	118	127
			Estimated calories burned per minute of activity based on an individual's body weight								
Activities		**lb**	120	140	160	180	200	220	240	260	280
Vigorous *(cont'd)*											
Skin diving			6.7	7.8	8.9	10.0	11.1	12.3	13.4	14.5	15.6
Skipping rope			7.7	9.0	10.2	11.5	12.7	14.0	15.3	16.5	17.8
Snowshoeing			10.6	12.3	14.1	15.8	17.5	19.3	21.0	22.7	24.4
Stair-climber machine			8.7	10.1	11.5	12.9	14.3	15.8	17.2	18.6	20.0
Step aerobics, 6-8 in. (15-20 cm) step			8.2	9.5	10.9	12.2	13.5	14.9	16.2	17.6	18.9
Swimming, lap, light or moderate effort			6.7	7.8	8.9	10.0	11.1	12.3	13.4	14.5	15.6
Swimming, leisure			5.8	6.7	7.7	8.6	9.6	10.5	11.4	12.4	13.3
Swimming, vigorous effort			10.6	12.3	14.1	15.8	17.5	19.3	21.0	22.7	24.4
Walking, 12 min per mi (1.6 km)			7.7	9.0	10.2	11.5	12.7	14.0	15.3	16.5	17.8
Walking with backpack			6.7	7.8	8.9	10.0	11.1	12.3	13.4	14.5	15.6
Weightlifting, vigorous effort			5.8	6.7	7.7	8.6	9.6	10.5	11.4	12.4	13.3

Based on selected MET values created by B.E. Ainsworth et al., 2000, "Compendium of physical activities: An update of activity codes and MET intensities," *Medicine and Science in Sports and Exercise* 32(9): S498-S504.

Appendix D
Forms for Progressing Toward an Active Lifestyle

Personal Time Study

Date: _____   Day of week: _____

Time slot	Tasks or activities	Physically active?	
		Yes	No
Midnight to 4:00 a.m.			
4:01 to 8:00 a.m.			
8:01 a.m. to noon			
12:01 to 4:00 p.m.			
4:01 to 8:00 p.m.			
8:01 p.m. to midnight			
Total time			

From S.N. Blair, A.L. Dunn, B.H. Marcus, R.A. Carpenter, and P. Jaret, 2011, *Active Living Every Day*, 2nd ed. (Champaign, IL: Human Kinetics).

Keeping Track of Thoughts

Week of _____

Instructions: Use this form to record the number of times you think about doing physical activity. Simply place a check mark in a box in section 1 each time you think about doing some physical activity. If you carry out your thoughts and do the activity you were thinking about, place a check mark in a box in section 2.

Keeping track of your thoughts about activity can help you start moving toward an active lifestyle.

Section 1	I thought about doing some physical activity.

Section 2	I carried out my thoughts and did the activity.

From S.N. Blair, A.L. Dunn, B.H. Marcus, R.A. Carpenter, and P. Jaret, 2011, *Active Living Every Day*, 2nd ed. (Champaign, IL: Human Kinetics).

Keeping Track of Physical Activity

Activity	Intensity level	2 min		10 min		Total min
Garden	Moderate	☐ ☐ ☐ ☐ ☐ ☐ ☐ ☐ ☐ ☐		☐ ☐ ☐ ☐ ☐ ☐ ☐ ☐ ☐ ☐		
	Vigorous	☐ ☐ ☐ ☐ ☐ ☐ ☐ ☐ ☐ ☐		☐ ☐ ☐ ☐ ☐ ☐ ☐ ☐ ☐ ☐		
Household	Moderate	☐ ☐ ☐ ☐ ☐ ☐ ☐ ☐ ☐ ☐		☐ ☐ ☐ ☐ ☐ ☐ ☐ ☐ ☐ ☐		
	Vigorous	☐ ☐ ☐ ☐ ☐ ☐ ☐ ☐ ☐ ☐		☐ ☐ ☐ ☐ ☐ ☐ ☐ ☐ ☐ ☐		
Leisure	Moderate	☐ ☐ ☐ ☐ ☐ ☐ ☐ ☐ ☐ ☐		☐ ☐ ☐ ☐ ☐ ☐ ☐ ☐ ☐ ☐		
	Vigorous	☐ ☐ ☐ ☐ ☐ ☐ ☐ ☐ ☐ ☐		☐ ☐ ☐ ☐ ☐ ☐ ☐ ☐ ☐ ☐		
Occupation	Moderate	☐ ☐ ☐ ☐ ☐ ☐ ☐ ☐ ☐ ☐		☐ ☐ ☐ ☐ ☐ ☐ ☐ ☐ ☐ ☐		
	Vigorous	☐ ☐ ☐ ☐ ☐ ☐ ☐ ☐ ☐ ☐		☐ ☐ ☐ ☐ ☐ ☐ ☐ ☐ ☐ ☐		
Sport	Moderate	☐ ☐ ☐ ☐ ☐ ☐ ☐ ☐ ☐ ☐		☐ ☐ ☐ ☐ ☐ ☐ ☐ ☐ ☐ ☐		
	Vigorous	☐ ☐ ☐ ☐ ☐ ☐ ☐ ☐ ☐ ☐		☐ ☐ ☐ ☐ ☐ ☐ ☐ ☐ ☐ ☐		
Stairs	Moderate (1 flight up = 10 steps)	☐ ☐ ☐ ☐ ☐ ☐ ☐ ☐ ☐ ☐		☐ ☐ ☐ ☐ ☐ ☐ ☐ ☐ ☐ ☐		
	Vigorous (4 flights up = 2 min vigorous work)	☐ ☐ ☐ ☐ ☐ ☐ ☐ ☐ ☐ ☐		☐ ☐ ☐ ☐ ☐ ☐ ☐ ☐ ☐ ☐		
Walking	Moderate	☐ ☐ ☐ ☐ ☐ ☐ ☐ ☐ ☐ ☐		☐ ☐ ☐ ☐ ☐ ☐ ☐ ☐ ☐ ☐		
	Vigorous	☐ ☐ ☐ ☐ ☐ ☐ ☐ ☐ ☐ ☐		☐ ☐ ☐ ☐ ☐ ☐ ☐ ☐ ☐ ☐		

From S.N. Blair, A.L. Dunn, B.H. Marcus, R.A. Carpenter, and P. Jaret, 2011, *Active Living Every Day*, 2nd ed. (Champaign, IL: Human Kinetics).

Step by Step: Weekly Activity Log

Week: _____

Daily step goal: _____   **Reward:** _____

Minutes-of-activity goal: _____   **Reward:** _____

Other goals: _____   **Reward:** _____

| Day of week | Date | Step goal | Actual steps | Min of activity | | Notes |
				Moderate	Vigorous	
Monday						
Tuesday						
Wednesday						
Thursday						
Friday						
Saturday						
Sunday						

Week: _____

Daily step goal: _____   **Reward:** _____

Minutes-of-activity goal: _____   **Reward:** _____

Other goals: _____   **Reward:** _____

| Day of week | Date | Step goal | Actual steps | Min of activity | | Notes |
				Moderate	Vigorous	
Monday						
Tuesday						
Wednesday						
Thursday						
Friday						
Saturday						
Sunday						

From S.N. Blair, A.L. Dunn, B.H. Marcus, R.A. Carpenter, and P. Jaret, 2011, *Active Living Every Day*, 2nd ed. (Champaign, IL: Human Kinetics).

Index

Note: The italicized *f* and *t* following page numbers refer to figures and tables, respectively.

About the Authors

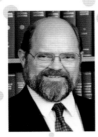

Steven N. Blair, PED, is a professor at the Arnold School of Public Health at the University of South Carolina in Columbia. His research focuses on the associations between lifestyle and health, with a specific emphasis on exercise, physical fitness, body composition, and chronic disease. As one of the most highly cited exercise scientists currently active in research, Dr. Blair has published more than 475 articles, chapters, and books in scientific and professional literature. He also was the senior scientific editor for the *U.S. Surgeon General's Report on Physical Activity and Health*.

Blair is a fellow of the American College of Epidemiology, Society of Behavioral Medicine, American College of Sports Medicine, American Heart Association, and American Academy of Kinesiology and Physical Education. He was also elected to membership in the American Epidemiological Society. He was the first president of the National Coalition for Promoting Physical Activity and is a past president of the American College of Sports Medicine and the American Academy of Kinesiology and Physical Education.

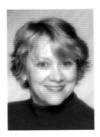

Andrea L. Dunn, PhD, is a senior scientist at Klein Buendel, Inc., a health communication research company in Golden, Colorado. She served as the project director and co-investigator of Project *Active*, ACT (Activity Counseling Trial), and PRIME (Physically Ready for Invigorating Movement Every day), all large-scale clinical trials involving sedentary adults. These studies helped sedentary adults learn behavioral skills vital for adopting and maintaining an active lifestyle. She has conducted public health research on physical activity interventions to improve a variety of health outcomes but particularly to improve mental health.

Dunn cowrote the curriculum for Project Active and PRIME that is the basis for Active Living Every Day. She has led intervention groups that tested the approach, and she is the lead author of the *Journal of the American Medical Association* article describing its efficacy.

Dunn has an MS in psychology and a PhD in exercise science and is a fellow of the American College of Sports Medicine and the Society of Behavioral Medicine.

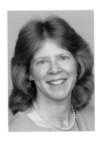

Bess H. Marcus, PhD, is Professor and Chair of the Department of Family and Preventive Medicine at the University of California, San Diego where she pursues research on physical activity and public health with funding from the National Institutes of Health. Dr. Marcus is a clinical health psychologist who has spent the past 25 years conducting research on physical activity behavior and has published more than 175 papers and book chapters as well as three books on this topic.

Dr. Marcus has developed a series of assessment instruments to measure psychosocial mediators of physical activity behavior and has also developed low-cost interventions to promote physical activity behavior in community, workplace, and primary care settings. Dr. Marcus uses a variety of channels to promote physical activity including print, telephone, and the Internet. Dr. Marcus has participated in panels for the American Heart Association, American College of Sports Medicine, Centers for Disease Control and Prevention, and National Institutes of Health; these panels have created recommendations regarding the quantity and intensity of physical activity necessary for health benefits. Dr. Marcus also does work examining the benefits of exercise for women who want to stop smoking. Marcus was a contributing author to the *Surgeon General's Report on Physical Activity and Health* and a member of the executive committee for the National Physical Activity Plan. Marcus served as an advisor on the curriculum development for the Cooper Institute's Project *Active* study that created *Active Living Every Day.*

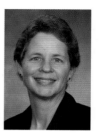

Ruth Ann Carpenter, MS, RD, is the founder and lead integrator at Health Integration, LLC. She was the cocreator of the curriculum and group cofacilitator for The Cooper Institute's Project *Active* study that created the Active Living Every Day program. Most recently she provided technical assistance and support during the testing of the 12-week version of the Active Living Every Day program.

Carpenter is a registered dietitian with a master's degree in applied nutrition and extensive coursework in exercise science. She has over 25 years of experience designing, developing, implementing, and evaluating nutrition and physical activity behavior change programs in community and worksite settings. She has coauthored six books and developed educational materials for clients such as the American Heart Association, Kellogg's, Roche, Tropicana, and Jenny Craig.

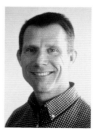

Peter Jaret is a medical journalist whose work has appeared frequently in the *New York Times, National Geographic, Reader's Digest, AARP Journal, Health, National Wildlife,* and other publications. He is the author of *Impact: From the Frontlines of Global Health* (National Geographic Books) and *Nurse: A World of Care* (Emory University Press).

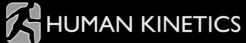
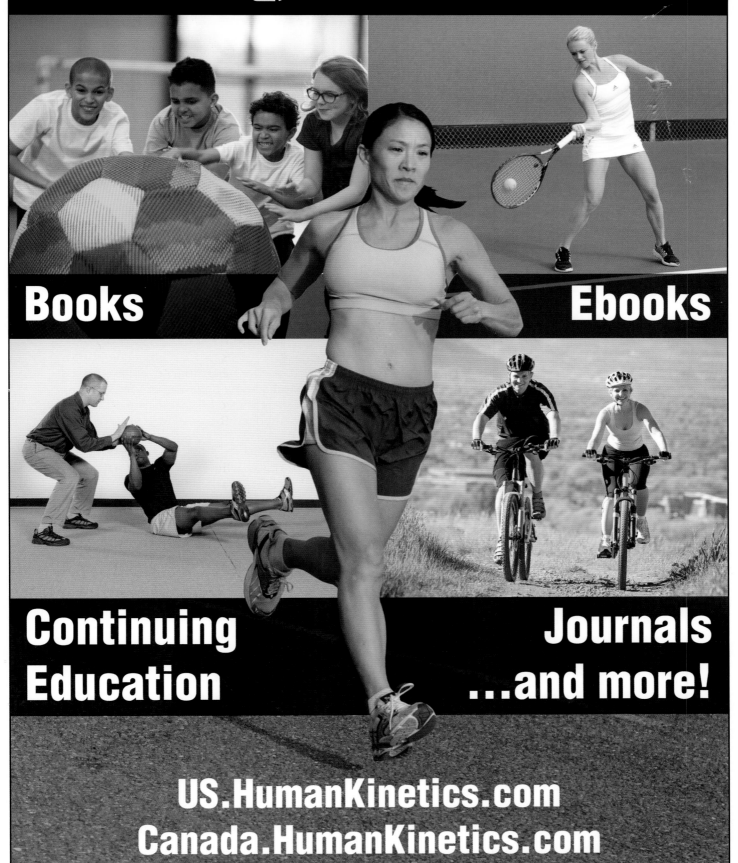